Physiotherapy for the Hip Joint

Physiotherapy for the Hip Joint

Dr. Patitapaban Mohanty

Associate Professor and Head, Department of Physiotherapy, Swami Vivekananda National Institute of Rehabilitation Training and Research, Olatpur, Bairoi, Cuttack

Monalisa Pattnaik

Assistant Professor, Department of Physiotherapy, Swami Vivekananda National Institute of Rehabilitation Training and Research, Olatpur, Bairoi, Cuttack

ELSEVIER

Publisher: Dolores Meloni
Acquisitions Editor: Belinda Kuhn
Editorial Project Manager: Pat Gonzalez
Project Manager: Kiruthika Govindaraju
Cover Designer: Matthew Limbert

3251 Riverport Lane
St. Louis, Missouri 63043

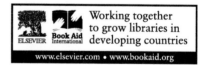

Working together to grow libraries in developing countries

www.elsevier.com • www.bookaid.org

Dedicated to
The Holy Budhha Bapa, Gurujee.
Without your blessings, we would not have been able to
achieve our goal.
P.P. Mohanty.
Monalisa Pattnaik.

Contents

About the authors

Dr. Patitapaban Mohanty, PhD (Medical science), has about 30 years of experience in teaching theoretical, practical, and clinical studies to Bachelor of Physiotherapy students and about 20 years of experience in teaching theoretical, practical, and clinical studies to Master of Physiotherapy students. Dr. Patitapaban Mohanty has more than 110 research publications in indexed national and international journals and is the author of 5 textbooks. Dr. Mohanty is a national accredited manual therapy teacher. His students are placed across the globe earning name and fame for the Institute. Dr. Mohanty is a PhD guide, member of the Board of studies, examiner, and paper setter of various universities across the country and editorial board member of a number of national and international journals.

Monalisa Pattnaik has about 30 years of teaching experience in theoretical, practical, and clinical studies to Bachelor of Physiotherapy students and about 20 years of teaching experience in theoretical, practical, and clinical studies to Master of Physiotherapy students. Mrs. Pattnaik has more than 110 research publications in indexed national and international journals and is the author of 5 textbooks. Mrs. Pattnaik serves as a guide to Master of Physiotherapy students, examiner, and paper setter of various universities across the country.

Preface

This book is written to meet the needs of students, academicians, and clinicians. The first chapter of *Physiotherapy of the Hip Joint* covers the basic anatomy and the biomechanics of the knee, knowledge of which is essential to understand the mechanical problems. Evaluation and assessment is the key for appropriate planning of the physiotherapy management of any problem, without which successful management may not be possible. We have tried our best to include as much evidence as possible. Almost all the hip problems related to physiotherapy are included, so that it will be convenient to get the overall physiotherapy management of the mechanical hip problems in one book. We hope this book will provide useful guidance to the students, teachers, and the clinicians. We have tried to give as much pictures as possible to understand the techniques easier.

The authors are having about 30 years of theoretical, practical, and clinical experiences and have tried their best to provide as much practical knowledge as possible. Any feedback from the students and academicians is welcomed to further improve the textbook.

We are thankful to Mr. Tapan Kumar Prusty, Niraj Kumar, Brahmananda Dash, and Ansuman Das for their assistance.

P.P. Mohanty

Monalisa Pattnaik

Anatomy and biomechanics

The hip is the most proximal of the lower extremity joints. Coxofemoral joint is the articulation of the acetabulum of the pelvis and the head of the femur (Fig. 1.1). It is a diarthrodial ball-and-socket joint that supports the weight of the head-arms-trunk (HAT) both in static erect posture and in dynamic postures such as ambulation, running, and stair climbing [1].

Bony components—hip is a synovial joint of ball and socket variety, formed by the articulation of acetabulum with head of femur. Normally, the acetabulum faces laterally, anteriorly, and inferiorly. Horseshoe-shaped articular surface is covered by the articular cartilage. The rough nonarticular portion of acetabular fossa is lined by fat-pad. Acetabular cavity encloses more than a hemisphere. It is deepened by fibro-cartilagenous acetabular labrum. It is difficult to pull the head from the acetabulum without removing or tearing acetabular labrum. Acetabular notch is traversed by transverse ligament of acetabulum, which converts the notch into a foramen. Acetabular artery, branch of obturator artery, eventually becomes artery of ligament of the head of femur passes through it.

The head of femur constitutes two-third of a sphere. The head is roughened slightly below and behind the center of the head known as fovea, to which ligament

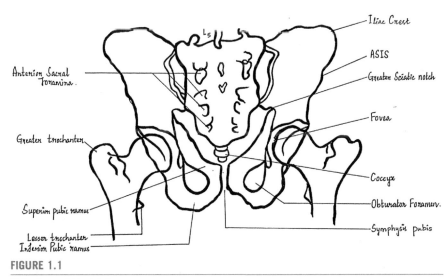

FIGURE 1.1

Osteology of hip joint.

Physiotherapy for the Hip Joint. https://doi.org/10.1016/B978-0-323-93649-1.00008-9

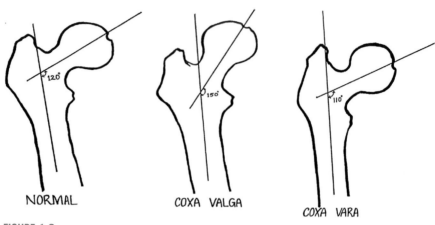

FIGURE 1.2

Neck shaft angle (angle of inclination).

of the head of the femur is attached [2]. The neck-shaft angle in the frontal plane is known as angle of inclination, which is about 150 degrees in newborn and gradually decreases to 125 degrees in adults. Persistent increase in neck-shaft angle is known as coxa-valga, and decrease in angle is known as coxa-vara [3] (Fig. 1.2).

Neck-shaft angle in transverse plane is referred as angle of torsion or angle of declination. Increase in neck shaft angle in the transverse plane is known as anteversion [3]. It is characterized by in-toeing gait. Decrease in torsonal angle is known as retroversion and one walks with out-toeing gait. Since, both the acetabulum and head of the femur face forward, a portion of head of femur remains uncovered by the acetabulum. A small area on posterosuperior aspect of head bears the load.

Greater trochanter is a prominence projecting laterally and superiorly from the junction of neck and shaft. Lesser trochanter lies posteromedially at the junction of neck and shaft. It provides attachment to iliopsoas muscle. Various muscles like hip abductor (Glutei) are attached to the outer aspect of G.T, and hip external rotators are attached to inner aspect of it to control the hip movements.

Trabecular pattern of upper femur reflects the normal stresses sustained by the hip. There are two sets of trabeculae (Fig. 1.3). The vertical bundles (medial trabecular system) travel straight upward from medial cortex of shaft of femur to the superior cortex of head, which resists vertical compressive force through the head of femur. The arcuate bundles (lateral trabecular system) run upward and medially from lateral cortex of shaft of femur to middle and inferior cortex of head of femur and resist bending moment [4]. There are two accessory (or secondary) trabecular systems of which one is considered compressive and the other is considered tensile. Secondary trabecular system runs from medial cortex at the base of neck upward laterally through the greater trochanter, which resists the tensile forces from the muscles attached to the trochanter. Another secondary trabecular system is confined to the trochanteric area femur. The areas in which the trabecular systems cross each other at right angles are areas that offer the greatest resistance to stress and strain. There is an area in the femoral neck in which the trabeculae are relatively thin

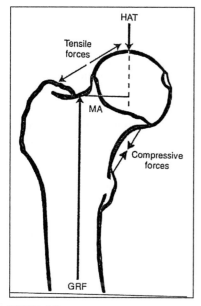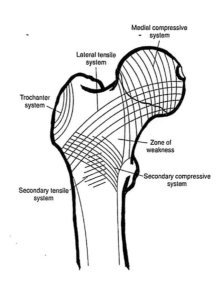

FIGURE 1.3

Trabecular pattern of the upper femur.

and do not cross each other-**ZONE OF WEAKNESS** [1]. The poor trabecular system at the neck makes it relatively weaker. It becomes weaker in elderly persons due to senile osteoporosis and in elderly female due to menopausal osteoporosis. So, fracture of neck of femur is one of commonest injuries seen in elderly persons that occur due to fall or stumbling due to imbalance.

Articular cartilage—the horse-shoe shaped area of acetabulum is covered by articular cartilage and the nonarticular portion of acetabular fossa is filled up by fat pad. The entire head except the fovea is covered by articular cartilage. Ligament of head of femur is attached to the fovea.

Capsule and ligaments—The articular capsule of the hip joint is an irregular, dense fibrous structure with longitudinal and oblique fibers. The capsule is attached proximally to the entire periphery of the acetabulum beyond the acetabular labrum. Fibers near the proximal attachment are aligned in a somewhat circumferential manner. The hip joint capsule is attached distally to intertrochanteric line anteriorly and about 1 cm proximal to intertrochanteric crest posteriorly [5]. Most of the portion of the neck is intracapsular. The joint capsule is reinforced by ilio-femoral ligament anteriorly. It is an inverted Y-shaped ligament that checks extension and internal rotation. It is thought to be the strongest ligament in our body. It allows the person to stand with the hip joint in extension using minimum or no muscle force (MF) by rolling the pelvis backward. A person hangs on the ligament. The person with paraplegia will able to stand by the support of ilio-femoral ligament. Ischio-femoral ligament become taught in extension and internal rotation. Pubo-femoral ligament become taught in adduction and internal rotation. Since all the ligaments become taught in extension—abduction—internal rotation; it is known as the closed pack for the hip joint [6]. The ligament of head of femur (ligamentus teres) becomes taught in adduction. Its function is relatively unimportant. The transverse ligament crosses the acetabular notch and converts it into a foramen through which the acetabular artery, a branch of obturator artery passes; eventually it accompanies the ligamentus teres.

Synovium—The synovium lines the joint capsule, acetabular labrum, fat pad present in the acetabular notch and the ligament of head of the femur. The intraarticular portion of neck of femur is lined by synovium. The synovial cavity of the hip joint often communicates anteriorly with the ilio-pectineal bursa.

Bursa—The ilio-pectineal bursa is the largest bursa present on the anterior aspect of hip joint underneath the iliopsoas muscle. It often communicates with the hip joint cavity. Therefore, persons with hip joint arthritis and synovitis complain of anterior hip pain and the effusion become prominent anteriorly. Laterally one or more trochanteric bursa is present underneath the glutei muscles over the greater trochanter. Posteriorly, ischial bursa is present underneath the hamstrings.

Blood supply—Head of the femur is supplied by nutrient artery, medial (posterior) and lateral (anterior) circumflex femoral arteries and artery accompanying ligamentum teres [7]. In case of synovitis, the intracapsular circumflex femoral arteries are compressed and blood supply to head of the femur is compromised. It may predispose to avascular necrosis of head of femur. Synovitis of hip joint may be one of the causes of the Legg-Calve-Perthes disease. In case of fracture neck of femur, both the circumflex femoral arteries and nutrient artery, intimately related to the neck may be damaged affecting the blood supply to head of femur. It leads to nonunion and avascular necrosis of head of femur. Higher is the fracture site more is the chance of damage to the arteries.

Nerve supply—The hip joint is supplied by branches of obturator nerve, superior gluteal nerve, nerve to quadratus femoris and branches of femoral nerve(L2-L1 segment).

Muscles—The role of the psoas major as a hip flexor is clear from its location anterior to the medio-lateral axis of hip that passes approximately through the center of the femoral head. Although it has a smaller moment arm (MA) for flexion than some other hip flexors such as the rectus femoris, sartorius, and tensor fasciae latae, its large physiological cross-sectional area (PCSA) makes it a strong hip flexor. According to one study of eight healthy young adults—resisted hip flexion while standing on the opposite limb recruits the psoas major more vigorously than other exercises and activities designed to elicit maximal contraction [8]. The center of mass of the HAT lies posterior to the flexion and extension axis of the hip joint, applying an extension moment to the hip. Contraction of the psoas major is able to produce a flexion moment to counteract the extension moment, but more recent EMG data reveal minimal activity (2% of maximum voluntary contraction) of the psoas major during quiet standing, which increases only slightly when standing in trunk hyperextension.

Weakness of the psoas major decreases the strength of hip flexion. Such weakness could produce difficulties in tasks such as lifting a limb in and out of the bath tub and climbing stairs. Although active hip flexion is an important element of normal locomotion, the amount of force required of the hip flexors during normal gait is relatively small. Therefore, slight-to-moderate weakness of the psoas major may have an imperceptible impact on locomotion. However, more severe weakness of the psoas major alters the late stage of the stance phase of gait when the hip flexors should accelerate the limb forward.

Tightness of the psoas major restricts hip extension range of motion (ROM). It may also limit trunk side-bending flexibility. In the upright posture, tightness of the psoas major is often manifested by increased lumbar extension. This posture results from the pull on the lumbar vertebrae toward the femur and simultaneous compensation of backward bending of the lumbar spine for the individual to keep the eyes on the horizon.

The iliacus is a large muscle with a PCSA equal to or greater than the PCSA of the psoas major. It is regarded with the psoas major as the primary hip flexor. Together, they are known as the iliopsoas muscle. The iliacus moves the hip joint directly and is an essential flexor of that joint. Because it attaches with the psoas major, the MA analyses at the hip are the same for the psoas major and iliacus. MA analysis suggests that the iliacus has little capacity to rotate the hip from the extended position and only a small advantage for lateral rotation once the hip is flexed [9].

Weakness of the iliacus decreases hip flexion strength. The functional effects are similar to those with weakness of the psoas major. However, the iliacus may be slightly active to prevent hip hyperextension in quiet standing.

The hip contains structures that can support the hip in quiet standing, even in the absence of muscular support. The anterior capsule with its three reinforcing ligaments provides passive limits to hip hyperextension. The subject who lacks muscular control at the hip can stand unsupported by assuming a position of hip hyperextension so that the weight of the HAT generates an extension moment at the hip. By resting in maximum hyperextension, the individual can use the passive support of the ligaments to prevent additional backward bending. This is known as Hanging on the ligaments.

Tightness of the iliacus reduces hip extension ROM. In the standing position, tightness of the iliacus results in an anterior pelvic tilt that is accompanied by hyperextension of the lumbar spine. As seen with a tight psoas major, a tight iliacus frequently leads to an increased lumbar lordosis [10]. If, however, the subject lacks hyperextension flexibility in the spine, tightness of the iliacus or psoas major can produce a forward lean and a flattened lumbar spine in upright posture. Bilateral hip flexion contractures are common and are an occupational hazard of office workers, truck drivers, and students, those who spend most of their day in sitting. It is not surprising to find hip flexion contractures in sedentary elders. However, individual variations in low back flexibility and strength can markedly affect the resulting compensations. Although stemming from the same musculoskeletal impairment, hip flexor tightness, the varied compensations produce different postural and functional presentations, often leading to disparate musculoskeletal complaints.

The individual with a flexible lumbar spine exhibits an excessive lumbar lordosis and may complain of pain from increased loads on the lumbar facet joints. The individual with diminished low back flexibility exhibits a flattened lumbar lordosis and forward lean that may lead to muscle strain and injury to the intervertebral disc from excessive loading. When only one hip has the contracture or when one hip has a larger contracture than the other hip, the effects on posture may vary. The important factor in unilateral hip flexion contracture is to determine which attachment site is more displaced. In case of femur been pulled towards the pelvis that effectively produces a shortened lower extremity, the patient can respond in a variety of ways to equalize the leg length. Compensations include dropping the pelvis ipsilaterally, plantar flexing the foot on the ipsilateral side, and flexing the knee on the ipsilateral.

The gluteus maximus is a large muscle with a PCSA at least 30% greater than that of the iliopsoas. It forms most of the contour of the buttocks. The function of the gluteus maximus as a hip extensor depends on the position of the body in space as well as the position of the hip joint itself. In the prone position, the gluteus maximus lifts the weight of the lower extremity to extend the hip with a concentric contraction. In quiet standing, because the HAT weight tends to extend the hip, the gluteus maximus is electrically silent. Mechanical analyses and computed tomography (CT) scans to examine the length of the MAs of the hip extensors from a position of 0 degrees of flexion to 90 degrees of flexion reveal that the MA of the gluteus maximus appears greatest around 0 degrees of flexion and decreases steadily to 90 degrees of flexion [11]. Other hip extensors, namely, the hamstrings and adductor magnus, reach their maximum MAs when the hip is more flexed. Weakness of the gluteus maximus results in decreased strength of hip extension and lateral rotation.

A classic gait pattern resulting from gluteus maximus weakness is known as the gluteus maximus lurch. The lurch is a rapid hyperextension of the trunk prior to, and continuing through, heel contact on the side of the gluteus maximus weakness. It has been suggested that the backward "lurch" moves the center of mass of the HAT weight to a position posterior to the hip joint, thus eliminating the need for the gluteus maximus to extend the hip.

Tightness of the gluteus maximus limits hip ROM in flexion and medial rotation. Athletes such as runners who have strongly developed gluteus maximus muscles can exhibit limited hip flexion ROM. Because hip movement is intimately related to low back movement, tightness of the gluteus maximus may produce excessive movement in the lumbar spine. Restrictions in hip flexion ROM can require an individual to use excessive trunk flexion during such activities as squatting to pick up an object from the floor or to tie a shoelace. Tightness of the gluteus maximus therefore may be a contributing factor to low back pain.

The broad proximal attachments of both the gluteus medius and gluteus minimus indicate that these muscles are quite strong and participate in functional activities that require considerable force. Although active abduction of the hip in an open chain is used in activities such as getting on and off a bicycle, the essential role of the abductor muscles occurs during closed chain activities such as walking and running. These activities of bipedal ambulation are characterized by intermittent periods of one-legged stance. During the time of single-limb support, the weight of the opposite limb and that of the HAT (the HAT-L weight) exerts an adduction moment on the stance hip, tending to make the body fall onto the unsupported side and adducting the hip on the stance side [12]. To hold the pelvis and the weight above it stable, the abductor muscles on the support side pull from their distal attachments on the femur to their proximal pelvic attachments. This pull, if strong enough, holds the pelvis level and prevents its dropping on the unsupported side. The ability to stabilize the knee and foot in three planes appears to depend, in part, on the alignment and stability of the hip. For example, as an individual steps down from a step or curb, she/he lowers body weight (BW) onto the lower step by flexing the weight-bearing hip and knee on the upper step. Inadequate stability of the weight-bearing hip appears to allow the weight-bearing knee to move into more valgus and the foot may pronate.

As single-limb support begins and the abductor muscles are too weak to hold the pelvis level, the HAT-L weight tends to cause the pelvis to drop on the unsupported side. Because this is a very unstable phenomenon and puts the subject at risk of falling, most subjects use a typical substitution. To avoid the pelvic drop on the unsupported side, the subject leans the trunk toward the supporting side. This lean moves the center of mass of the HAT-L weight to the lateral aspect of the hip joint on the stance side. In this position, the HAT-L weight no longer tends to adduct the hip, thus eliminating the need for active abduction force. The resulting gait pattern is so characteristic of hip abductor weakness that it is dubbed as gluteus medius limp, although it is likely to involve both the gluteus medius and the gluteus minimus.

Trendelenburg Test is a simple clinical screening procedure for abductor weakness and uses single-limb stance and the postural compensation present with abductor weakness. The test is known as the Trendelenburg test and uses quiet, single-limb standing. It is positive for abductor weakness on the stance side when the subject leans excessively toward the stance limb or when the pelvis drops on the unsupported side. Preliminary evidence suggests that a positive Trendelenburg test indicates considerable weakness of the abductor muscles.

Abductor tightness, although not common, does exist. Tightness of these muscles results in decreased ROM in adduction and, perhaps, in lateral rotation. Such tightness is found in individuals with arthritis whose position of comfort frequently includes hip flexion and abduction. The functional consequences of an abduction contracture are seen most often in upright posture and may include changes in pelvic alignment to maintain erect posture or in the positions of the other joints of the lower extremity to optimize the base of support.

Adductors of the hip—Despite the areas of disagreement surrounding the individual actions of the adductor muscles, most investigators agree on one important functional role of the adductors to stabilize the pelvis during weight shifting from one limb to the other [13]. This role is seen during gait as the adductors contract during the transitions from stance to swing and swing to stance. The adductors also help stabilize the hip during squatting activities. In squatting to lift something from the floor, an individual typically has the hips slightly abducted. Inspection of the ground reaction force (GRF) reveals that it produces an abduction moment at the hip that must be countered by an adduction moment produced by contraction of the adductor muscles. Anyone who has gardened can probably verify the adductor muscles' role by recalling the muscle soreness in the inner thighs after the garden cleanup or long gardening time.

Adductor weakness is not common but may result from an injury to the obturator nerve. Such injuries have been reported following surgeries such as laparoscopic or endoscopic prostatectomies and even rarely following vaginal deliveries. Symptoms include gait instability and an abducted gait in which the affected limb contacts the ground with the hip excessively abducted.

Tightness of the adductors is relatively common and may result from adaptive changes in muscles that are not routinely stretched. Such tightness is likely in sedentary individuals or in individuals on bed rest who do not receive active or passive exercises. In addition, adductor muscles are commonly affected by central nervous system disorders resulting in spasticity. Examples of such disorders include cerebral vascular accidents (strokes), multiple sclerosis, and cerebral palsy. In an ambulatory individual, extreme tightness of the adductors of the hip can create significant problems in gait, leading to scissors gait. During swing, the limb with the tightness may have difficulty passing the stance limb, causing the individual to trip over the stance limb. The limb with the tightness also may land in front of the opposite limb at the beginning of double-limb support, again presenting a threat of tripping. Spasticity of the hip adductors is a common clinical finding in individuals with cerebral palsy [14].

In children, adductor spasticity is an important contributing factor to hip dislocation and hip dysplasia. At birth, the normal alignment of the femur is valgus directing the femoral head toward the superior aspect of the acetabulum when the hip is in the neutral position. Adduction from the neutral position moves the femoral head laterally in the acetabulum. Because the acetabulum is shallowest at birth, prolonged positioning of the hip in adduction can sublux or dislocate the hip joint. The presence of spasticity of the adductors presents significant additional risk for dislocation, and surgical release of spastic muscles around the hip, including the adductors, reduces the dislocating forces, helping to minimize the incidence of dislocation and hip dysplasia.

Because the gluteus maximus is the strongest of the hip lateral rotators, weakness of the short lateral rotators may be difficult to detect. The traditional position in which to test hip lateral rotation strength is seated with the hip and knee flexed. In sitting, the gluteus maximus' lateral rotation MA is shortened; however, its muscle length is increased [15]. In contrast, the lateral rotation MAs for the quadratus femoris and obturator externus are lengthened with the hip flexed, but the MAs of the other short lateral rotators are shorter. There is no position in which to isolate the contributions of the short lateral rotators from the gluteus maximus. This also means that there is no single position in which to strengthen the short lateral rotators. Like weakness, isolated tightness of the short lateral rotators may be hard to observe. However, the proximity of the sciatic nerve to these muscles, particularly to the piriformis, which may even be pierced by the nerve, makes tightness of these muscles clinically relevant. If tight, these muscles may exert pressure on the sciatic nerve, producing pain radiating into the lower extremity.

The piriformis syndrome refers to pain associated with tightness or spasm of the piriformis muscle that puts pressure on the underlying sciatic nerve, causing radicular symptoms similar to signs of disc pathology. The symptoms can be aggravated by stretching or contracting the piriformis, that is, by medially rotating the hip passively to stretch the muscle or by resisting lateral rotation, causing the piriformis to contract. The clinician uses passive or resisted movements to elicit the patient's symptoms and to identify piriformis syndrome. The classic stretch for the piriformis muscle is hip flexion with adduction and medial rotation even though research shows that in hip flexion the piriformis is a medial rotator. Research suggests that sitting with the knees crossed combining hip flexion with adduction and lateral rotation applies a significant stretch to the piriformis [16].

Unlike the other actions of the hip, there are no muscles at the hip whose primary and consistent action is medial rotation of the hip. The gluteus medius and minimus are capable of medial rotation of the hip, particularly when the hip is flexed. The gluteus maximus and piriformis also may contribute to medial rotation of the hip when the hip is flexed. Some of the hip adductors may generate small medial rotation moments, but their contributions are small and variable. Another muscle described as a medial rotator of the hip is the tensor fasciae latae. The medial hamstrings, the semimembranosus, and semitendinosus also exhibit small medial rotation MAs with the hip in extension. These data reveal that the muscles that medially rotate the hip depend on hip position and are intimately related to the function of the knee. The most common functional use of active medial rotation of the hip occurs during the stance phase of gait when the pelvis rotates over the fixed femur and as the hip moves from the flexed to the extended position. During this period, the abductors contract to support the pelvis in the frontal plane, and the hamstrings are supporting the hip and knee in the sagittal plane. Their activity in medial rotation demonstrates an efficient use of muscles to perform simultaneous tasks.

Janda (1987) classified the skeletal muscles on the basis of evolution and development into two functional groups—tonic (postural) and phasic (motion) [17]. Umphred et al. (2001) identified that the tonic muscles are involved in repetitive rhythmic activity and are activated in flexor synergies, whereas phasic muscles work against gravity and are activated in extensor synergies [18]. Tonic muscles consist of predominantly type I fibers (slow twitch), whereas phasic muscles consist of predominantly type II fibers. Tonic muscles are fatigue resistant, whereas phasic muscles get fatigue easily. Tonic muscles have a natural tendency to shorten, whereas phasic muscles have a tendency to lengthen and become weak. Nerve impulses reach the postural muscles before the phasic muscles, so the postural muscles inhibit the antagonistic phasic muscles. Tight prone postural muscles become tighter and weak prone phasic muscles become weaker. Muscle imbalance leads to joint dysfunction and poor movement pattern. Thus, hip flexors, back extensors become tight and abdominals, hip extensors become weaker resulting in lower cross syndrome. Pectorals, upper trapezius, levator scapulae become tight and neck flexors, rhomboids, serratus anterior become inhibited and weak resulting into upper crossed syndrome.

Biomechanics—In normal standing position the toes face outward by about 10−15 degree and foot angle is about 30 degrees, patellae face straight forward. In the normally aligned pelvis, the ASISs of the pelvis lie on a horizontal line with the PSIS and on a vertical line with the symphysis pubis.

The hip joint is intrinsically very stable. Acetabular cavity encloses the head of the femur to provide bony stability. The acetabular labrum further deepens the acetabular cavity reinforcing the stability. With the acetabular labrum intact, it is difficult to pull the head out of acetabulum. Hip joint being one of the larger joints, it is subjected to atmospheric pressure equal to 25 kg, which is sufficient to maintain the stability. With all the soft tissues around the joint removed, the weight of the limb can be freely supported. It drops down by making a drilled hole through the acetabulum. The joint capsule is reinforced by various ligaments that provide static stability. Twisting of the ligaments pull the joint into close packed position in extension—internal-rotation and abduction. It is referred as screw home movement of the hip joint. It is the most stable and congruent position.

Both head of femur and acetabulum face forward in normal standing position. So, their axis is not coincidental. There are two positions in which the axis becomes coincidental and joint becomes stable. One is close pack position (extension-abduction-internal rotation) that is, in standing and the other one is hip flexion to 90 degrees, slight abduction and slight external rotation, that is, in quadruped position.

There is a relatively small area of contact between acetabulum and femoral head that bears the weight. In standing or upright weight-bearing activities at least **half** the weight of the HAT (the gravitational force) passes down through the pelvis to the femoral head, whereas the **GRF** travels up the shaft. These two forces, nearly parallel and in opposite directions, create a force couple with a MA equal to the distance between the superimposed BW on the femoral head and the GRF up the shaft. These forces create a **bending moment** (or set of shear forces) across the femoral neck [19]. The bending stress creates a tensile force on the superior aspect of the femoral neck and a compressive stress on the inferior aspect. A complex set of forces prevents the rotation and resists the shear forces that the force couple causes; among these forces are the structural resistance of two major (medial and lateral) trabecular systems and three minor trabecular systems (secondary tensile system, secondary compressive system, and trochanteric system).

Since the load bearing area is relatively small, degeneration of the hip joint occurs overtime. At mid-stance phase of gait cycle, the hip joint is in full extension (close pack position), so the load over the head of femur is relatively less as the area of contact is more. Persons with hip flexion deformity, fails to attain the close pack position and transfer the load in semiflexed position, which is incongruent. As the load over head of the femur increases due to reduced contact area, one is likely to develop early degenerative joint disease.

Since hip joint is intrinsically stable, normal hip joint rarely dislocates. Hip is more prone to dislocate in a position of flexion, abduction, internal rotation as the ligaments are laxed and joint is noncongruent. Dislocation of hip occurs in case of dash board injury, collapse of roof of coal mines on stooping workers.

Hip joint has three degrees of freedom. Flexion-extension occurs in sagittal plane and coronal axis, abduction-adduction occurs in coronal plane and sagittal axis, medial and lateral rotations occur in transverse plane and vertical axis. Range of hip flexion is about 120–140 degrees, which is limited by contact between front of the thigh with the abdomen. Extension range is about 20–25 degrees and is limited by the tension of ilio-femoral ligament. Hip flexion-extension range can be measured in supine lying at the edge of the bed or in side lying position with the axis at the tip of greater trochanter. It can be confirmed by abducting and adducting the hip. Abduction is about 40–50 degrees and limited by the contact of greater trochanter with the pelvis bone or tension of hip adductor muscles. Adduction is limited by the contact with the opposite thigh and tension of capsule-ligamentous structures. Range is about 30 degrees. Axis for abduction—adduction movements is the junction of lateral two-third and medial one-third of the line joining ASIS and symphysis pubis or about half inch below the mid-inguinal line. Range of hip external rotation is about 50–60 degrees and that of internal rotation is about 40–50 degrees. Medial rotation is limited by the tension of joint capsule or hip external rotators, whereas lateral rotation is limited by the femoral anteversion. As the femoral retroversion decreases and anteversion increases, internal rotation range proportionate increases at the cost of external rotation range. The axis of hip rotation in high sitting or prone lying with the knee flexed to 90 degree is the center of patella tibio-femoral joint line at the apex of patella and the fixed arm remains horizontal and movable arm along the long axis of tibia [20]. Hip joint is freely movable in all the planes; therefore, soft tissue injury around the hip joint is relatively uncommon. Any force acting on hip joint may cause movement without injury. As it is connected to longer lever arms of the femur as well as the entire extremity, the impact gets multiplied that may cause some soft tissue injury.

During normal human locomotion hip joint is about 30 of flexion at heel strike following which it extends, becomes neutral at mid-stance phase of gait cycle and then hyper-extends. It starts flexing following heel off, becomes neutral at mid-swing and 30 of flexion at subsequent heel strike. Flexion is required for chair sitting, for sit to stand and for step climbing.

In single leg standing (Fig. 1.4 a) whole body except the supporting extremity is the lever, hip joint of the supported side is the fulcrum (F), effort (E) is provided by the hip abductors of the supported side, BW passing through the line of gravity that passes in front of the center of gravity present in front of the S2 vertebra generate a moment that tends to rotate the pelvis on the unsupported side downwards. Downward pelvic tilt on the unsupported side is checked by the upward moment created by the contraction of supported side hip abductors. While standing on right side BW creates clockwise moment, which is counter-balanced by the anticlockwise moment created by the hip abductors of the right side. The supported side hip abductors work

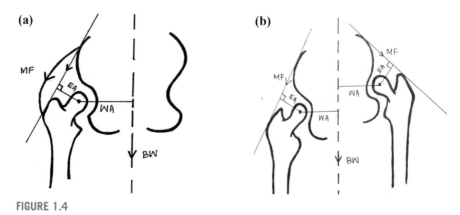

FIGURE 1.4

Loading of the hip joint in single leg standing (a) normal, (b) in case of limb length descrepancy.

with reverse origin and insertion to prevent dropping of pelvis on unsupported side. Similarly, during single leg standing on left side BW creates anticlockwise moment, which is counter-balanced by the clockwise moment created by the left hip abductors. Hip abductors MF acts along the line of muscle pull, that is, line joining origin to insertion applies the effort (E) and the effort arm (EA) is its perpendicular distance. Weight arm (WA) is the perpendicular distance of the weight line from the fulcrum. From cadaveric study, it has been found that WA is equal to double the EA (WA = 2 EA). In balanced state, the clockwise moment is equal to the anticlockwise moment. The equation becomes, MF x EA = BW x WA. Replacing WA by 2 EA, MF x EA = BW x 2 EA → MF = 2BW

So to support the BW in single leg standing, the hip abductors on the supported side has to work with the force equal to double the BW.

In single leg standing, supported side hip abductors work isometrically with reverse origin and insertion. Since there occurs no movement, hip abductors MF acts over the joint as joint compressive force. So, the hip joint is subjected to load equal to BW and hip abductor MF. Load = BW + Abductor MF (2BW) = 3BW. In single leg standing supported side hip joint is subjected to three times BW load. One Kg increase in BW adds 3 kg more load to the hip joint during single stance phase of each gait cycle.

In case of LLD (Fig. 1.4b) stands erect either by flexing the longer side hip and knee bearing almost all the weight on the shorter side, or by plantar flexion of the shorter leg bearing almost all the weight on the longer side. In standing with pelvic tilt either due to true and/or apparent pelvic tilt, line of gravity shifts toward the shorter side. WA for the lower side decreases and that on higher side increases.

During single standing on the shorter side, the weight line shifts toward the shorter side. Thus, the WA on the shorter side is reduced and that on the longer side is increased than the normal. The equation become, MF x EA = BW X WA (WA< 2EA). Hip abductor MF to prevent downward drop of the pelvis on unsupported side will be < 2BW. So, the load over the hip of the shorter side will be < 3BW. While standing on the longer side, the equation becomes MF x EA = BW X WA (WA >2 EA). Hip abductor MF to balance the pelvis will be > 2BW and the load on the longer side hip will be > 3BW. Increased loading on the longer side hip joint during each stance phase of the gait cycle predisposes it to degenerative joint disease.

While using walking stick on the affected side (Fig. 1.5a) one transfers some BW through the walking stick. The GRF passing through the walking stick and upper extremity creates a moment that tends to rotate the pelvis downwards around the supported hip joint toward the unsupported sound side. The perpendicular distance of the stick from the hip joint is the lever arm (GA). Both the BW (BW X WA) and GRF (GRF X GA) create moments in same direction that tends to rotate the pelvis downwards on the unsupported side. To counter-balance it, hip abductors on the affected (supported) side have to act generating moment (MF X EA) in opposite direction. There is extra burden on the hip abductor mechanism to support the moment generated by the GRF. So, it is in a disadvantage state.

In Balanced state the equation becomes, MF x EA= (BW x WA) + (GRF x GA), here, GA = MA of the GRF passing through the walking aid that create a moment in the direction of moment created by BW. Now, hip abductor has to work to a greater extent to balance the moment generated by both the weight and GRF. The load over the affected hip joint is equal to BW + hip abductors MF, which will be greater than the normal load (Fig. 1.5).

While using walking stick on the sound side (Fig. 1.5b) one transfers some BW through the walking stick. The GRF passing through the walking stick and upper extremity creates a moment that tends to rotate the pelvis downwards around the supported hip joint toward the sound side that in turn elevates the pelvis on the unsupported side. Both the hip abductors (MF X EA) and GRF (GRF X GA) create moments in same direction that tends to rotate the pelvis upwards on the unsupported side to counter-balance the moment generated by the BW (BW X WA) tilting the pelvis downwards on the unsupported side. The hip abductor mechanism is

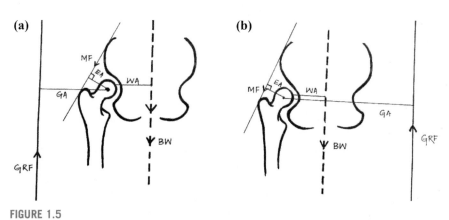

FIGURE 1.5

Biomechanics of single stick (a) on the affected side, (b) on the unaffected side.

supported by the GRF. So, it is in an advantage state. In Balanced state the equation becomes (MF x EA) + (GRF x GA) = (BW x WA). Now, hip abductor has to work to a lesser extent to balance the moment generated by the weight. The load over the affected hip joint will be lesser than the normal load. Thus, use of walking stick on the opposite side is recommended in case of unilateral hip pathology.

Persons with hip pathology usually walk with lurching (lateral trunk bending) on the affected side during loading phase of gait cycle and the Trendelenburg's sign is positive. During the loading phase, the hip joint is subjected to BW (BW) and hip abductor MF amount of load. The BW of the individual cannot be reduced; the EA of the hip abductor mechanism of the individual also remains constant. The load over the hip joint can be reduced by minimizing hip abductor activity. One leans toward the affected side during the loading phase of gait cycle and shift weight line toward the hip joint (Fulcrum). Thus, the WA gets reduced and to balance the moment, generated by BW (BWxWA), hip abductor muscle activity reduces proportionately (MF X EA). More one leans toward the affected side, proportionately hip abductor activity reduces and the load over the hip joint (BW + MF) also reduces. Excessive leaning toward the affected side, so that weight line passes through the hip joint and WA becomes zero. Now, one can walk without using hip abductors.

Lurching gait occurs if there is any abnormality in the lever system. Problem in the fulcrum itself i.e., hip arthritis, increase in BW, problem in the effort, that is, hip abductors weakness, abnormality in EA, that is, reduced EA as in case of Coxa-valga, hip abductors are in disadvantageous state as in case of coxa-vara, etc. conditions may result in lurching gait. In case of pain in the hip joint, one tries to reduce the load bearing through the hip joint while standing and walking. So, one drags the sound limb with short step to avoid/minimize load bearing on the affected hip and takes a larger step as a compensatory means on the affected side. This is referred as antalgic gait (Fig. 1.6).

Anterior and posterior pelvic tilt is motions of the entire pelvic ring in the **sagittal plane around a coronal axis.** [21] In the normally aligned pelvis, the ASISs of the pelvis lie on a horizontal line with the PSIS and on a vertical line with the symphysis pubis. Normal pelvic alignment in sagittal plane is maintained by the balance between hip flexors-back extensors and hip extensors—abdominals force couples. Imbalance in force couples results in pelvic tilt in saggital plane. Anterior and posterior tilting of the pelvis on the fixed femur produces hip flexion and extension, respectively. Hip joint extension through posterior tilting of the pelvis brings the symphysis pubis up and the sacrum of the pelvis closer to the femur, rather than moving the femur posteriorly on the pelvis. Hip flexion through anterior tilting of the pelvis moves the ASISs anteriorly and inferiorly; the inferior sacrum moves farther from the femur, rather than moving the femur away from the sacrum.

Lateral pelvic tilt is a frontal plane motion of the entire pelvis around an antero-posterior axis [21]. In the normally aligned pelvis, a line through the ASISs is horizontal. Pelvis may tilt downward (Pelvic Drop) or upward (Pelvic Hike) on the frontal plane. Shortening of hip abductors produces infra pelvic tilt, whereas hip adductors shortening produces supra pelvic tilt (Fig. 1.7).

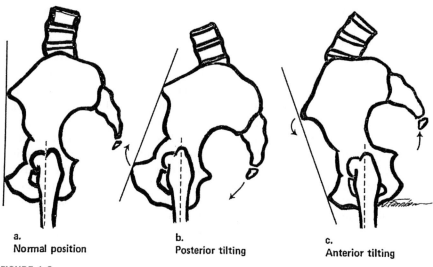

| a. | b. | c. |
| Normal position | Posterior tilting | Anterior tilting |

FIGURE 1.6

Pelvic tilt.

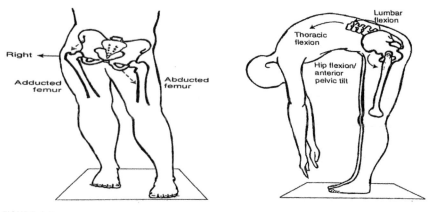

FIGURE 1.7

Lateral pelvic tilt.

Lateral Shift of the Pelvis—If both limbs are weight bearing, lateral tilt of the pelvis will cause the pelvis to shift to one side or the other. With pelvic shift, the pelvis cannot hike but can only drop. Because there is a closed chain between the two weight-bearing feet and the pelvis, both hip joints will move in the frontal plane in a predictable way as the pelvic tilt (or pelvic shift) occurs. If the pelvis is shifted to the right in bilateral stance, the left side of the pelvis will drop, the right hip joint will be adducted, and the left hip joint will be abducted.

Anterior and posterior pelvic rotation: Pelvic rotation is motion of the entire pelvic ring in the transverse plane around a vertical axis [21]. Forward rotation of the pelvis occurs in unilateral stance when the side of the pelvis opposite to the supporting hip joint moves anteriorly. Forward rotation of the pelvis produces medial rotation of the supporting hip joint. Backward rotation of the pelvis occurs when the side of the pelvis opposite the supporting hip moves posteriorly. Posterior rotation of the pelvis produces lateral rotation of the supporting hip joint. Pelvic rotation can occur in bilateral stance as well as unilateral stance, as is true for lateral pelvic tilt. If both feet are bearing weight and the axis of motion occurs around a vertical axis through the center of the pelvis, the terms forward rotation and backward rotation must be used by referencing a side, for example, forward rotation on the right and backward rotation on the left. Pelvi-femoral motion can increase the range of forward flexion of the head and arms by combining hip flexion, anterior pelvic tilt, and flexion of the lumbar spine. This combination permits the hands to maximize the reach toward the ground. When the femur, pelvis, and spine move in a coordinated manner to produce a larger ROM than is available to one segment alone, the hip joint is participating in what will predominantly (but not exclusively) be an open-chain motion termed pelvi-femoral motion. During forward bending, spine moves cephalo-caudally followed by sacral nutation (forward nodding—sacral base moves antero-inferiorly and apex moves postero-superiorly), then anterior rotation of pelvis. During extension, innominates move first for posterior rotation of pelvis, then sacral counter-nutation (backward nodding—sacral base moves postero-superiorly and apex moves antero-inferiorly), and at last spine extends caudal-cephally.

References

[1] Levangie PK, Norkin CC. The hip complex. In: Joint structure and function: a comprehensive analysis. 4th ed. F.A. Davis Company; 2005. p. 355—94.

[2] Lo D, Talkad A, Sharma S. Anatomy, bony pelvis and lower limb, fovea capitis femoris. In: StatPearls [internet]. Treasure Island (FL: StatPearls Publishing; 2021. PMID: 30085547.

[3] Zaghloul A, Mohamed EM, Maaty MT, El-Adl El-Saied G, Hammad A. Computing measurements of femoral neck shaft angle in children and adolescents from nile delta. Orthoped Rheumatol Open Access J 2020;17(1):19—25.

[4] Hertling D, Kessler RM. Hip. Management of common musculoskeletal disorders: physical therapy principles and methods. 4th ed. Lippincott Williams and Wilkins; 2005. p. 443.

[5] Singh V. Hip joint. Textbook of anatomy abdomen and lower limb. 2nd ed. Elsevier India; 2014. p. 377—86.

[6] Thorp LE. Hip anatomy. In: Nho S, Leunig M, Larson C, Bedi A, Kelly B, editors. Hip arthroscopy and hip joint preservation surgery. New York, NY: Springer; 2015. https://doi.org/10.1007/978-1-4614-6965-0_113.

[7] Zaghloul A, Mohamed EM. Hip joint: embryology, anatomy and biomechanics. Biomed J Sci Tech Res 2018;12(3):9304—18.

[8] Neumann DA. Kinesiology of the hip: a focus on muscular actions. J Orthop Sports Phys Ther 2010;40(2):82—94.

[9] Sajko S, Stuber K. Psoas Major: a case report and review of its anatomy, biomechanics, and clinical implications. J Can Chiropr Assoc 2009;53(4):311−8.

[10] Siccardi MA, Tariq MA, Valle C. Anatomy, bony pelvis and lower limb, psoas major. In: StatPearls. Treasure Island (FL): StatPearls Publishing; 2021. PMID: 30571039.

[11] Németh G, Ohlsén H. In vivo moment arm lengths for hip extensor muscles at different angles of hip flexion. J Biomech 1985;18(2):129−40.

[12] Ganvir SD, Ganvir S, Nagarale AV. Biomechanics of hip joint. Biomechanics of joints. 1st ed. Jaypee Publishers; 2013.

[13] Dubey L, Karthikbabu S, Mohan D. Effects of pelvic stability training on movement control, hip muscles strength, walking speed and daily activities after stroke: a randomized controlled trial. Ann Neurosci 2018;25(2):80−9.

[14] Goyal V, Laisram N. Grading of adductor spasticity in cerebral palsy − a new approach. Indian J Phys Med Rehabil 2015;26(1):2−5.

[15] Hogervorst T, Vereecke EE. Evolution of the human hip. Part 2: muscling the double extension. J Hip Preserv Surg 2014;2(1):3−14.

[16] Lowe W. The paradoxical piriformis: stretching for the hips. Massage Today; 2019. https://www.massagetoday.com/articles/1576162523411/Stretching-for-the-Hips.

[17] Janda V. Muscles and motor control in low back pain: assessment and management. In: Twomey LT, editor. Physical therapy of the low back. New York: Churchill Livingstone; 1987. p. 253−78.

[18] Gibbons J. Sacroiliac joint stability, muscle imbalances, and the myofascial slings. Functional anatomy of the pelvis and the sacroiliac joint: a practical guide. North Atlantic Books; 2017.

[19] Rudman KE, Aspden RM, Meakin JR. Compression or tension? The stress distribution in the proximal femur. Biomed Eng Online 2006;5:12.

[20] Loudon JK. Biomechanics and pathomechanics of the patellofemoral joint. Int J Sports Phys Ther 2016;11(6):820−30.

[21] Lewis CL, Laudicina NM, Khuu A, Loverro KL. The human pelvis: variation in structure and function during gait. Anat Rec 2017;300(4):633−42.

Evaluation

Hip joint is supplied by L2-S1 segments. Typically, a person with hip pathology complains of pain on the anterior aspect of the thigh up to the front of the knee. Pain is more experienced on the front of the knee (L3 segment). Usually, in children with poor history, it is often confused as knee pathology. Pain on the front of thigh may refer from the thoraco-lumbar spine. Pain from hip pathology is more experienced on the front of the hip joint. Lateral hip pain may be due to trochanteric bursitis [1]. Pain on the posterior aspect of the hip joint could be radiating from lumbar spine, referred from SI joint, piriformis syndrome etc.

Since hip joint is freely movable in all the planes, acute traumatic pathology is rarely seen. Hip joint is often the site of degenerative joint disease as it is subjected to about 3 times BW compressive load over a relatively smaller area of head of the femur during loading phase of each gait cycle. In new born, Congenital dislocation of hip (CDH), 5–10 years of age perthes disease, at adolescent slipped capital femoral epiphysis, elderly persons degenerative joint disease (OA) and tuberculosis may occur at any age. Elderly person with history of fall may sustain fracture neck of femur [2]. Incidence of fracture trochanter is rather relatively more than fracture neck of femur. Therefore, the clinician should take thorough history followed by detailed physical examination to determine the pathology. To exclude radiating pain from the spine or referred pain from SI joint, detailed history is helpful. Prior to physical examinations screening test may be performed to rule out spine, SI joint pathology.

The screening includes active physiological movements followed by passive terminal overpressure in all possible directions. If all the movements are found to be full in range and free from reproducing the original symptom, the joint is excluded having the pathology.

History

- Mode of onset—sudden or insidious
- Elderly persons with history of fall, found inability to get up and bear the load could be due to fracture neck of femur. Groin pain of sudden onset is due to strained hip adductors [3]. Pain and spasm of hip flexor and adductors with limitation of movement and antalgic gait could be due to arthritis.

- Asymmetry in the limb length in new born could be due to CDH joint. Insidious onset of limping during 1st decade could be due to perthes disease [4].
- Sudden traumatic limping in adolescent or gradual onset of limping associated with obesity in adolescent is due to slipped capital epiphysis.
- Hip pain of gradual onset and limping in elderly person occurs from degeneration.

Physical examination
Observation
1. GAIT
   - Lurching to affected side is suggestive of hip abductor weakness or pain in hip.
   - Dropping of pelvis on unsupported side may occur due to weakness of hip abductor on the opposite side [5].
   - Backward trunk bending or increased lumbar lordosis is due to hip extensor weakness or hip flexors contracture.
   - Persistent inclination of pelvis to one side during all phase of gait cycle is suggestive of hip abductor or adductor contracture [6].
2. FUNCTIONAL ACTIVITIES
   - Inability to sit erect or sacral sitting is suggestive of loss of hip flexion range. One finds difficulty to lean forward to remove the shoes, socks, and trousers due to limitation of hip flexion range.
3. GENERAL POSTURE and BODY BUILT
   - Ectomorphic (lean and long)
   - Mesomorphic (muscular and well built)
   - Endomorphic (Big and Fat)

Inspection
1. Skin—No skin changes could be seen in case of hip pathology as the hip joint is deep seated, hip pathology may not be reflected at the skin level.
2. Soft tissue—
   - Wasting of glutei may be present.
   - Swelling—Hip joint effusion is not usually detectable from outside as the hip joint is deep enough. It may be visible on the front of hip as the swelling/effusion communicates through ilio-pectineal bursa [7].
3. Bony landmark—Check the following bony landmarks-Malleoli, tibial tuberosity, patella, femoral condyle, GT, ASIS, Iliac crest, PSIS, spine of vertebrae, tip of shoulder, etc.

Check the relationship with each other to find out any abnormality. Normally lateral malleolus is downward and backward to medial malleolus, medial femoral condyle is downward to lateral femoral condyle, ASIS is leveled with PSIS, tip of GT lies on the line joining ASIS and ischial tuberosity. Deviation shows abnormality. Find out the relationship of two identical bony landmarks on both the sides from a reference point, that is, ground in standing and any point on midline of body (Xiphisternum, Umbilicus, symphysis pubis) in lying position for bilateral symmetry. Suppose from malleolus to GT are bilaterally symmetrical and GTs are not leveled. It indicates something wrong between GT and ASIS. May be fracture neck of femur, coxa valga, coxa vara, dislocation, or arthritis.

From the front inspect whether the patient stands straight, comfortable, symmetrical, shoulder level, bears equal weight on both the sides, hip abduction/adduction, pelvic obliquity, level of ASIS, patella position, foot position, thigh wasting, skin for scar, trophic changes, etc.

From the back inspect whether the patient stands straight, comfortable, symmetrical, shoulder level, scoliosis, bears equal weight on both the sides, hip abduction/ adduction, pelvic obliquity, level of PSIS, gluteal fold, popliteal fold, Gluteal wasting, skin for scar, heel position, etc.

From the side inspect the patient's lumbar lordosis, hip knee flexion, scar, recent bruising, sinus, wasting, etc.

Movement evaluation

Persons with hip pathology often complain of pain during weight bearing activities therefore hip movements should be evaluated in weight bearing position [8]. Active physiological nonweight bearing movements may not reproduce the original symptom.

1. **Active weight bearing physiological movements**—Standing, single-leg standing (Trendlenberg, Fig. 2.1), squatting, single-leg mini-squat, running and jumping, cross leg sitting, cross sitting.
2. Active nonweight bearing physiological movements—
   - Check the range, pain response, crepitus, willingness, strength, painful arc, etc. pain may not be reproduced except in acute spasmodic condition.
   - Hip movements are compensated by movement of pelvis and lumbar spine, so the original symptom may not be reproduced.
3. Passive physiological movements—
   - Hip movements are compensated by the movements of pelvis and lumbar spine. Hip deformities are almost always transferred to the pelvis and lumbar spine [9]. Therefore, square/level the pelvis and bring the lumbar spine to neutral position so that original hip deformity can be determined/estimated.
   - Passive physiological movements of hip joint can be checked in supine lying position or in side lying.

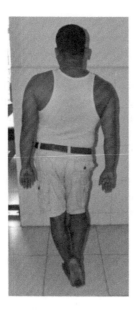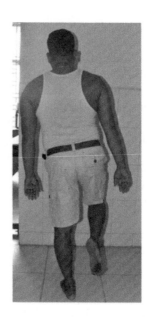

FIGURE 2.1

Trendlenberg test.

- Check hip flexion with knee flexed.
- Check hip flexion with knee straight to find out length of hamstring muscle.
- Bilateral hip abduction—adduction is checked in supine lying with knee straight as well as with knee in flexion to differentiate the shortening of long adductors from short adductors.
- Bilateral rotation of hip should be check in prone with knee flexed to 90 degrees, so that the pelvis remains fixed, trunk rotation can be prevented and movements on both the sides can be compared.
- Check hip extension in side lying with opposite hip and knee in full flexion or in prone lying.
- Note the range, pain, end feel, crepitus, painful arc, etc.
- To check hip flexion-extension ROM, with the pelvis fixed in neutral position, Thomas test has to be performed in case of increased lumbar lordosis and anterior pelvic tilt [10].

  Thomas Test—(Fig. 2.2) Subject is in sit lying position instead of supine lying in the presence of knee flexion deformity. Flex the opposite hip and knee to reduce increased lumber lordosis, if the thigh on affected side is raised off the couch, the test is said to be positive, suggestive of hip flexor shortening.

  Most of the cases even with complete hip and knee flexion, the increased lumbar lordosis doesn't reduce back to normalcy. It requires modification of the test. Flex both hips and knees to restore normal lumbo-pelvic alignment.

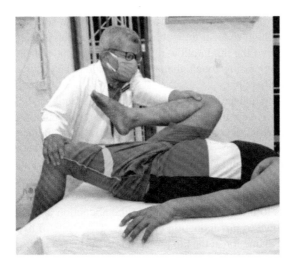

FIGURE 2.2

Thomas test.

With the sound hip and knee flexion maintained, extend the affected hip till the pelvis tends to tilt forward. Measure the flexion deformity by goniometer.

The further modification of Thomas test is as follows:

- Limitation of hip adduction suggest tensor fascia lata (TFL)shortening
- Limitation of internal rotation suggest iliopsoas shortening
- Limitation of knee flexion suggests rectus femoris shortening.

In case of infrapelvic tilt which is often seen in case of hip abductor shortening

Ober's Test—(Fig. 2.3) Subject is in side lying position on the sound side with hip and knee in flexion. Therapist stands behind with one hand over the

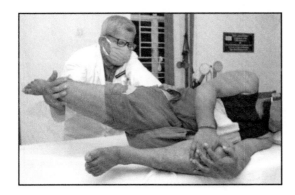

FIGURE 2.3

Ober's test.

pelvis and other around the bend knee with forearm supporting the leg. Abduct the thigh to level the pelvis and with the pelvis fixed in neutral position extend the thigh, allow the thigh to drop down. If the thigh fails to fall on the supporting couch, then the test is said to be positive, suggestive of TFL shortening [11].

In case of hip abductor tightness, one bends the trunk to the affected side to bring the foot in contact with the ground. As a result, the affected side pelvis tilts downwards. In case of infrapelvic tilt, to square the pelvis in supine lying, abduct and hyper-abduct the thigh, till the pelvis is leveled. Abduction occurs in the hip joint without changing the position of the pelvis. At the end range, GT comes in contact with the pelvis and with hyper abduction pelvis is pushed upward. Fix the pelvis by one hand and adduct the thigh till the ASIS tends to tilt downward. Measure the abduction angle by goniometer which is equal to hip abduction deformity. The range of hyper-abduction beyond the abduction at the hip joint tends to correct the infrapelvic tilt is the amount of hip abduction deformity.

Supra-pelvic tilt is often due to ipsilateral hip adductors shortening [12]. In case of hip adductors shortening, one side bends the trunk to opposite side in order to keep the foot flat on the ground and legs parallel. Adduct and hyper adduct the thigh beyond the midline till the pelvis is leveled. Adduction of the hip joint will not alter the state of the pelvic tilt. Hyper-adduction will pull the upwardly displaced pelvis downward. With one hand fix the pelvis in leveled state, and abduct the thigh till ASIS tends to move upward. Measure the amount of adduction deformity by goniometer.

Straight leg raising—(Fig. 2.4) With the pelvis fixed it is usually performed to measure the length of hamstring muscle. In supine lying, fix the pelvis by

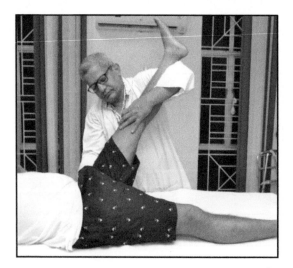

FIGURE 2.4

Straight leg raising.

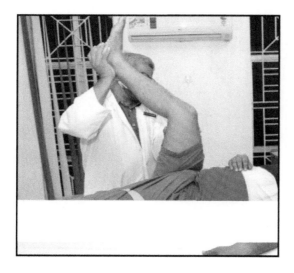

FIGURE 2.5

Alternately.

one hand, with other hand on the front of knee and forearm support the leg, raise the leg straight upward. Most of the time fixation of the pelvis is found to be difficult by this method. To overcome this difficulty, opposite hip may be fixed in extension and internal-rotation position. Alternately it can be done in side lying position.

Alternately (Fig. 2.5), hamstring length can be checked in 90-90 SLR in supine lying position. Flex the hip to 90, fix the thigh by one hand, and then extend the knee, measure the angle short of full knee extension [13]

4. **Passive joint play**—Check the AP, PA glide of head of femur over acetabulum, lateral distraction, caudal/longitudinal glide. Note the amplitude and pain response by comparing it with sound side in identical joint position.

AP glide—(Fig. 2.6) In supine lying or in sidelying. AP glide can be checked with hip flexed to 90 and knee in full flexion by applying pressure through the bend knee along the long axis of femur.

In supine or sidelying position, place the thenar eminence over the front of the greater trochanter and push it backward by using the body weight.

PA glide—(Fig. 2.7) Prone lying or side lying, place the thenar eminence over the back of the greater trochanter and push it forward by using the body weight.

Lateral distraction—It is checked in supine lying by fixing the pelvis by one hand and using a belt placed around the groin as high as possible on the medial aspect of the thigh and therapist's waist, pull the head of the femur out by moving the pelvis backward.

Longitudinal/caudal glide—It can be checked in supine lying by pulling the leg downward, grasping above malleoli or grasping proximal to knee joint or pushing above the GT in caudal direction.

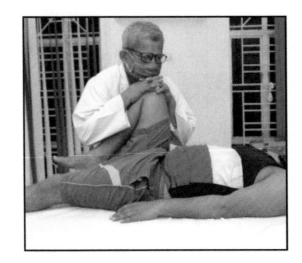

FIGURE 2.6

AP glide.

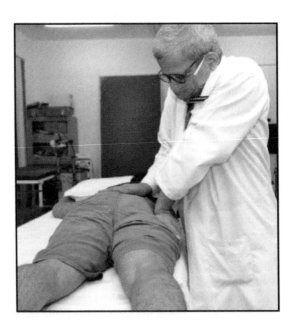

FIGURE 2.7

PA glide.

5. **Resisted isometric test**—Check the strength and pain response by comparing it with other side in identical joint position.
   - Hip flexor—pain suggests iliopectineal bursitis or sprain of iliopsoas/tendinitis
   - Hip extension with knee straight, apply resistance at ankle-pain at origin may be due to Ischial bursitis. Pain on upper part of thigh is due to hamstring strain.
   - Hip adductors are checked bilateral symmetrically suggests adductors/Rider's Strain.
   - Hip abductors can be tested bilateral symmetrically, and pain may be due to trochanteric bursitis or Gluteus medius tendinitis.
   - Hip rotators can be checked in prone lying with the knee flexed to 90 degrees by applying bilateral symmetrical resistance around ankle and foot.
   - Resisted hip abduction with hip flexed to 60 is suggestive of piriformis syndrome [14].

Neuromuscular evaluation

- Sensation
- Motor—tone, strength/voluntary control
- Reflexes—DTR, superficial reflexes
- Autonomic—bowel-bladder, pulse, temp, sweating, BP, etc.

Palpation

1. Skin—Check for temperature, texture, moisture and mobility. Rise in temperature, moist, smooth, glossy, shiny erythematous skin suggest increased vascularity, may be due to acute inflammation (vascular phenomenon) or acute reflex sympathetic dystrophy (sympathetic dysfunction)
2. Soft tissue—Check the swelling, wasting of soft tissue. To estimate the amount of swelling or wasting, girth measurement at particular level by using flexible measuring tape can be done and compare it with the same at the identical level on opposite side. To differentiate between intraarticular and extraarticular swelling, fluctuation test is performed. Since hip joint is a very deep joint, fluctuation test may not be informative. Continuity, consistency, mobility, etc. of various anatomical structures can be tested.
3. Bony landmark—
   - Relationship with each other—Check various bony landmarks such as navicular tubercle, medial and lateral malleoli, tibial tubercle, patella, femoral condyles, greater trochanter, ASIS, PSIS, iliac crest, spinous processes, tip of the shoulder, mastoid process, etc. on the affected side to

determine normal relationship between two bony land marks from the knowledge of surface anatomy. It may be disturbed in case of fracture, fracture mal-union, dislocation, dysplasia.

- Relationship from reference point in standing, ground is taken as reference where as in lying, any bony land mark on the midline/manubrium sternum, xiphi-sternum, umbilicus, symphysis pubis may be taken as reference.
- Check two identical bony landmarks on both the sides find out their bilateral symmetrical distances from the reference point. Symmetry upto a particular bony landmark on both the sides and asymmetry of the two identical bony landmarks above it indicate abnormality (shortening, fracture mal-union) between the two.

Special test

1. ORTOLANI and BARLOW'S (Fig. 2.8)—Both are performed in new born with CDH. Child is in crook lying. Therapist grasps the bent thigh with the thumb on medial aspect of femur as high as possible and fingers on GT. Abduct the thighs till resistance to movement is felt, try to push the head of femur into the acetabular cavity by using the fingers. A click sound may be produced and determine further abduction movement will be possible suggestive of reduction of dislocated hip. This is referred as Ortolani test [15]. Adduct the thighs, using the thumb try to push the head of the femur out of the acetabular cavity. A click sound suggests dislocation of hip is known Barlow test [16].

2. BRYANT's TRIANGLE—(Fig. 2.9) Subject in supine lying, draw a parallel line from ASIS on the couch, the second horizontal line is drawn from tip of GT parallel to the first line. Join ASIS to tip of GT to close right-angled

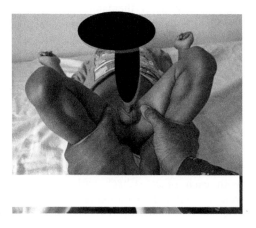

FIGURE 2.8

ORTOLANI and BARLOW'S.

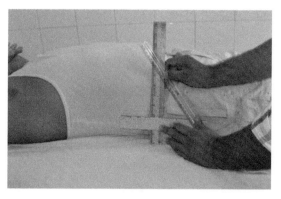

FIGURE 2.9

BRYANT's TRIANGLE.

triangle. Measure the length of horizontal line, which indicates the supra-trochanter length of femur. Compare it with the opposite side, reduced length suggest dislocation, coxavara, osteo-arthritis of hip joint, fracture neck of the femur, etc. increased length is suggestive of coxavalga.

3. NELATON's LINE—(Fig. 2.10) In sidelying position, join ASIS to the ischial tuberosity. Normally, the tip of GT lies on spino-ischial line. TIP of GT lies above the line in case of CDH, Coxavara and below the line in case of cox-avalga [17].

4. SCHOEMAKER's LINE—(Fig. 2.11) Join tip of GT with ASIS and extend it normally it bisects the midline at the level of umbilicus. It bisects the midline

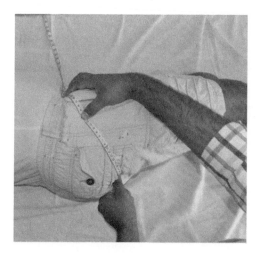

FIGURE 2.10

NELATON's LINE.

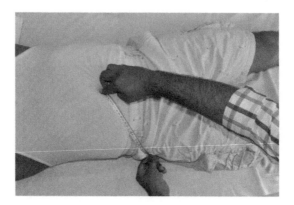

FIGURE 2.11

SCHOEMAKER's LINE.

below the umbilicus in case of CDH, coxavara and above the umbilicus in case of coxavalga.

5. **TELESCOPIC TEST** (Piston or Dupuytren's Test)—Subject in supine lying. Fix the pelvis by one hand with the index finger over the tip of GT. With the hip flexed to 90 and knee flexed, grasp around the bend knee by other hand, apply axial distraction and compression along the long axis of the femur. Compare it with the other side excessive movement suggest joint laxicity/subluxatable.

6. **TRENDLENBERG'S SIGN**—

Fig. 2.12 Subject in standing position, check the level of both ASIS by placing the thumbs over it. Ask the subject to bend the affected knee with the trunk

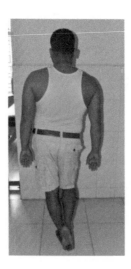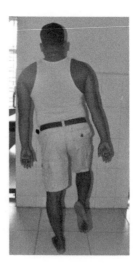

FIGURE 2.12

TRENDLENBERG'S SIGN.

straight. Repeat the same on the affected side, dropping of the pelvis downward on the unsupported unaffected side suggest the test is +ve indicating defect in the level system, that is, weakness of hip abductors, pain in hip joint, reduced effort arm as in case of coxavalga too much increase in body weight, dislocation of hip, coxavara, etc. [18]

7. THOMAS'S TEST—(Fig. 2.13) Subject in sit lying, bent the sound hip and knee till the increased lumbar lordosis is reduced to normal. If the thigh on the affected side is raised off the couch, the test is positive. Sometimes, with full flexion of hip and knee, the lumbar lordosis is not reduced to normal and it requires modification of the test. Flex both the hips and knees till the lordosis is reduced to normal, with the sound hip and knee fixed in flexion, extend the affected hip, and measure the hip flexion deformity by goniometer.

   Further modification can be done:
   - Limitation of hip adduction—TFL tightness
   - Limitation of hip internal rotation—Iliopsoas tightness
   - Limitation of knee flexion—Rectus femoris

8. OBER'S TEST—(Fig. 2.14) Subject in side lying position and therapist stands behind. Therapist's one hand is placed over lateral aspect of pelvis and other hand support the bent knee with leg supported over forearm. Abduct the thigh to level the pelvis. Fix the pelvis and allow the leg to drop down. If the limb remains in hanging position, the test is positive suggestive of hip abductors shortening. Limitation of hip extension adduction—TFL shortening. Limitation of HIP adduction with knee flexion/extension—IT band shortening.

9. PIRIFORMIS TEST—(Fig. 2.15) Subject in side lying with test leg uppermost. Patient flex the test hip 60 degree with knee flexed. Stabilize the hip with one hand and apply a downward pressure to knee. If piriformis is tight, pain is elicited in muscle. If piriformis pinching the sciatic nerve, pain results in

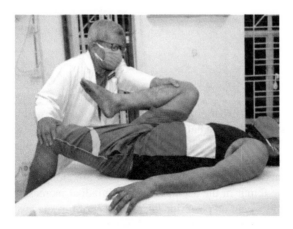

FIGURE 2.13

THOMAS'S TEST.

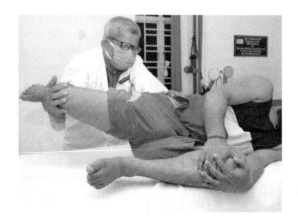

FIGURE 2.14

OBER'S TEST.

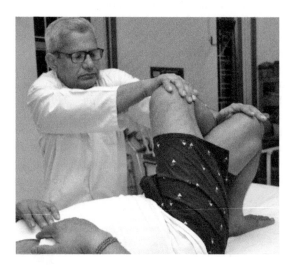

FIGURE 2.15

PIRIFORMIS TEST.

buttock and patient experience sciatica. Resisted lateral rotation with the muscle on stretch (hip medially rotated) can cause the same sciatica.

10. SCOURING—(Fig. 2.16) Subject in supine lying. Flex the hip to 90 and knee in full flexion. Therapist fixes the pelvis by one hand and other hand is placed over bend knee reinforced by chin. Apply pressure along long axis of femur and rotate the femur in the acetabulum with gradual increase in flexion and adduction angle. Pain on posterior-lateral aspect of hip suggests shortening of posterior-lateral hip joint capsule. Click sound may be produced during maneuver suggest OA [19].

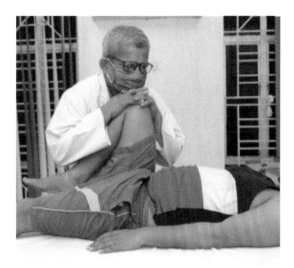

FIGURE 2.16

SCOURING.

11. ELY's TEST—(Fig. 2.17) Subject in prone lying if the pelvis is raised off the couch which increased in lumbar lordosis suggest iliopsoas tightness knee flexion increases the lumbar lordosis suggest rectus femoris tightness.

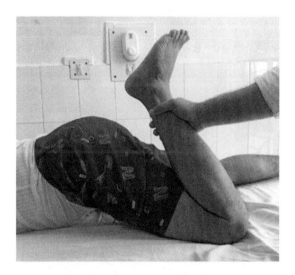

FIGURE 2.17

ELY's TEST.

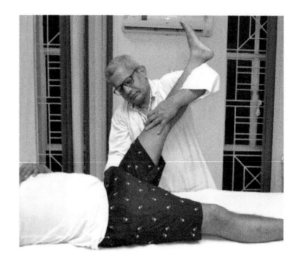

FIGURE 2.18

SLR.

12. SLR—(Fig. 2.18) In supine lying position, fix the pelvis by one hand, with other hand on the front of knee and forearm support the leg, raise the leg straight upward. Most of the time fixation of the pelvis is found to be difficult by this method. To overcome this difficulty, opposite hip may be fixed in extension and internal rotation position.

13. HIP 90-90 SLR—(Fig. 2.19) Fix the femur with hip flexed to 90 degrees with the pelvis fixed, extend the knee and measure the deficiency in the angle from straight knee 20 degrees lack of knee extension is considered as normal.

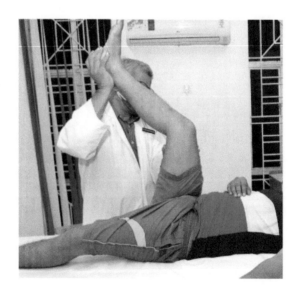

FIGURE 2.19

HIP 90-90 SLR.

14. PHELPS TEST—Subject in prone with knee extended. Abduct both the legs as far as possible. The knees are then flexed to 90 degrees, try to abduct further. If abduction further increases, gracilis contracture is there.
15. NOBLE's COMPRESSION TEST—Subject in side lying/supine lying. Hip and knee flexed to 90 degrees. Thumb pressure is applied lateral to femoral epicondyle and slowly extends the knee passively. Severe pain at about 30 degrees of knee extension suggests IT band friction syndrome [20].
16. BAER's SACROILIAC POINT—is tender in case of SI joint lesion or iliacus spasm. This point lies approximately 2 inches from the umbilicus on an imaginary line drawn from ASIS to the umbilicus.
17. CRAIG's TEST—(Fig. 2.20) For femoral anteversion-subject in prone lying, flex both the knees to 90 degrees and perform bilateral hip internal rotation increase in hip internal rotation range at the cost of external rotation is suggestive of femoral anteversion. Increase in external rotation range at the cost of internal-rotation would be due to femoral retro-version [21].
18. POSTERIOR LABRAL TEAR TEST—Subject in supine with full hip flexion, adduction and medial rotation. Take the hip into extension combined with abduction and lateral rotation. Groin pain, pt.'s apprehension, or the reproduction of patient's symptoms, with or without a click suggestive of posterior labral tear, anterior hip instability or posterio-inferior impingement. Also called as apprehension test if apprehension occurs toward the end of ROM during test [22].

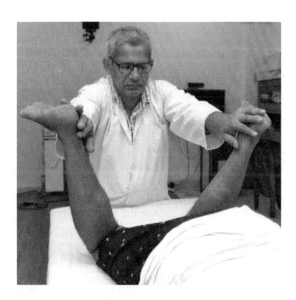

FIGURE 2.20

CRAIG's TEST.

19. FULCRUM TEST—Subject sits with knees bent over the edge of bed with feet dangling. Place the arm under the pt.'s thigh acts as a fulcrum. Fulcrum arm is moved from distal to proximal along the thigh as gentle pressure is applied by therapist to the dorsum of knee. If stress # is present, pt. complains of sharp pain and express apprehension when the fulcrum arm is under the # site [23]. Bone scan confirms the diagnosis.
20. GALEAZZI SIGN (ALLIS TEST)—Subject in supine with both hips and knees flexed. If one knee is higher than the other test is +ve. Good for assessing unilateral CDH/DDH. Children from 3 to 18 month.
21. MEASUREMENT OF LEG LENGTH—
22. Apparent leg length—Supine lying with both the limbs parallel with each other and in line with the trunk. Measure the length from xiphi-sternum or umbilicus to tip of medial malleolus or sole of heel with foot in neutral position and compare the both.
23. True Limb Length—Subject in supine lying. Square/level the pelvis. In case of infrapelvic tilt, abduct, and hyperabduct the thigh till ASIS on both the side are leveled. With pelvis leveled, adduct the thigh till the ASIS on the affected side tends to drop down. Position the sound limb in identical position. Take the measurement from ASIS to tip of medial malleolus or sole of heel with foot in neutral position and compare it with sound side [24].
24. Segmental Limb Length—Subject in crook lying. Femoral length is measured from tip of GT to lateral femoral epicondyle. Tibial length is measured from medial tibial flare to tip of medial malleolus. Supratrochanteric length of femur is measured by Bryant's triangle.

Diagnostic imaging

Standard AP and axial (lateral/frog-leg) views are taken.

- AP view (Fig. 2.21) shows Neck-shaft angle(coxa vara/valga), Shape of femoral head, Femoral head uncovering, Head tear drop distance, abnormal neck, offset (flattening of superior femoral head) is called pistol grip deformity [25], Joint spaces, Presence of osteophytes or arthritis, Presence of any bony disease, any evidence of fracture or dislocation, evidence of pelvic distortion, pelvic lines, and other landmarks.
- Shenton's line is curved drawn along the medial curved edge of the femur and continuing upward in a smooth arc along the inferior edge of the pubis. Broken line is indicative of dislocation or fracture. Disruption of pelvic ring indicates severe injury. Hilgenreiner line is a horizontal line drawn between inferior parts of ilium [26], Perkins's line is a vertical line drawn through upper outer points of the acetabulum, Acetabular index/Hilgenreiner angle is a line from the lateral to medial edge of acetabulum and angle formed by two lines called as acetabular/

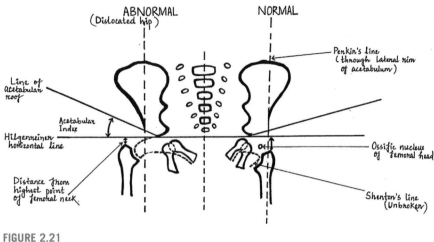

FIGURE 2.21

AP view.

hilgenreiner angle [27]. Greater the slope, lesser the stability of femoral head in acetabulum. Acetabular index normal 30 degrees.

- Ossific nucleus of femoral head should be in the inner lower quadrant. If lies in upper outer quadrant, indicative of DDH. In newborn ossification center is not visible. In DDH head of femur and acetabulum both may be affected. Acetabular index will be more than 30 degrees on affected side.
- Sagging rope sign seen in AVN of developing head. It indicates damage to growth plate with marked metaphyseal reaction and severe disease process.
- Tear drop sign—Migration of femoral head upward in relation to pelvis caused by degeneration as seen in OA, may be detected by this sign.
- Head at risk sign with leg calve perthes disease, cage's sign, calcification lateral to epiphysis, lateral migration of head (increased inferiomedial space), angle of epiphyseal line (horizontal), metaphyseal reaction. Patient who exhibits three or more head at risk sign have a poor prognosis so surgery is indicated.

Axial/Lateral/Frog Leg View—Patient lies supine with flexion, abduction, and lateral rotation of hip. This view provides a true lateral view of head and neck. First view shows slipping of head any pelvic distortion may also be seen.

- Sagging rope sign in leg calve perthes only femur head is affected but damage of growth plate due to avascular necrosis indicate severe disease process and sagging rope sign may be seen [28].
- Tear drop sign in OA due to degeneration, migration of femoral head in relation to pelvis may be detected by tear drop sign. Tear drop is visible at the base of pubic bone, extending vertically downward to terminate in a round tear drop or head. A line is drawn between the two tear drops and extended to the femoral heads on both sides. We can measure from the tear drop to femoral head. More

than 10 mm difference between two sides indicates significant migration of head.

Head at risk sign in leg calve perthes we can note the following head at risk signs:

- Cage's sign—a small osteoporotic segment on the lateral side of epiphysis that appears to be translucent.
- Calcification lateral to the epiphysis (if collapse is occurring).
- Lateral subluxation of head (an increase in the inferomedial joint space).
- Angle of epiphyseal line.
- Metaphyseal reaction.
- Patient's having three or more head at risk signs have a poor prognosis and surgery is needed.

Sign's of Slipped Capital Femoral Epiphysis—Widened epiphyseal line, Lipping or stepping may see as occur in lateral films, superior femoral neck lines does not transect the overhanging ossified epiphysis, Shenton's line does not exhibit continuous arc [29]. In addition to Slipped Capital Femoral Epiphysis causing a coxa vara, fracture or congenital malformations can lead to same deformity.

Arthrography may indicate a possible inverted limbus (infolding of a meniscus like structure) or a hour glass configuration from a contracted capsule. In CDH to show where the unossified femoral head lies relative to labrum. If hip cannot be reduced following dislocation, arthrography needed.

CT Scan is indicated specially for bony abnormality, for example, anteversion, retroversion, size and shape of head and acetabulum. In new born lack of ossification limits its use.

MRI is indicated specially for soft tissue like bursitis, tendon lesion as well as osseous tissue—osseous necrosis, femoral neck stress #, labral tear). It is excellent for congenital abnormalities. It is used as examination of choice for the evaluation of unexplained hip pain.

Scintigraphy (bone Scan) helps the diagnosis of stress fracture, necrosis and tumor.

Ultrasonography is a nonirradiation technique used to detect hip abnormalities like soft tissue problems, for example, swelling.

References

[1] Shbeeb MI, Matteson EL. Trochanteric bursitis (greater trochanter pain syndrome). Mayo Clin Proc 1996;71(6):565—9.
[2] Thorngren KG, Hommel A, Norrman PO, Thorngren J, Wingstrand H. Epidemiology of femoral neck fractures. Injury 2002;33(3):1—7.
[3] Serner A, Weir A, Tol JL, Thorborg K, Roemer F, Guermazi A, Yamashiro E, Hölmich P. Characteristics of acute groin injuries in the adductor muscles: a detailed MRI study in athletes. Scand J Med Sci Sports 2018;28(2):667—76.

[4] Santili C, Júnior WL, Goiano Ede O, Lins RA, Waisberg G, Braga Sdos R, Akkari M. Limping in children. Rev Bras Ortop 2015;44(4):290−8.

[5] Gandbhir VN, Lam JC, Rayi A. Trendelenburg gait [Updated 2021 Aug 19]. In: Stat-Pearls [Internet]. Treasure Island (FL): StatPearls Publishing; January 2022. Available from: https://www.ncbi.nlm.nih.gov/books/NBK541094/.

[6] Metaxiotis D, Accles W, Siebel A, Doederlein L. Hip deformities in walking patients with cerebral palsy. Gait Posture 2000;11:86−91.

[7] Tatu L, Parratte B, Vuillier F, Diop M, Monnier G. Descriptive anatomy of the femoral portion of the iliopsoas muscle. Anatomical basis of anterior snapping of the hip. Surg Radiol Anat 2001;23(6):371−4.

[8] McCarthy JC, Busconi BD, Owens BD. Assessment of the painful hip. In: Early hip disorders. New York, NY: Springer; 2003.

[9] Ike H, DorrL TN, Stefl M, McKnight B, Heckmann N. Spine-pelvis-hip relationship in the functioning of a total hip replacement. J Bone Jt Surg 2018;100(18):1606−15.

[10] Schache AG, Blach PD, Murphy AT. Relation of anterior pelvic tilt during running to clinical and kinematic measures of hip extension. Br J Sports Med 2000;34:279−83.

[11] Puniello MS. Iliotibial band tightness and medial patellar glide in patients with patello-femoral dysfunction. J Orthop Sports Phys Ther 1993;17:144−8.

[12] Husson JL, Mallet JF, Huten D, Odri GA, Morin C, Parent HF. The lumbar-pelvic-femoral complex: applications in hip pathology. Orthoped Traumatol 2010;96(4): S10−6.

[13] Surve DJ, Nikam PP. Effect of dynamic stretching warm-up protocol on hamstring flex-ibility in roller-skaters: an experimental study. Indian J Publ Health Res Dev 2019; 10(11):76−80.

[14] Kirschner JS, Foye PM, Cole JL. Piriformis syndrome, diagnosis and treatment. Muscle Nerve 2009;40(1):10−8.

[15] Lee KY, Yun EJ. Hip ultrasound in the neonates; the meaning of click sound on Ortolani test. J Kor Soc Ultrasound Med 1997;16(3):265−9.

[16] Jones DA. Neonatal hip stability and the Barlow test. A study in stillborn babies. J Bone Jt Surg Br 1991;73(2):216−8.

[17] Kamath BJ, Saraswati V, Bansal A, Pai V. Clinical evaluation of hip joint in sagittal plane using pelvifemoral angle. J Clin Orthop Trauma 2013;4(4):171−3.

[18] Hardcastle P, Nade S. The significance of the Trendelenburg test. J Bone Jt Surg Br 1985;67(5):741−6.

[19] Lee S, Nardo L, Kumar D, Wyatt CR, Souza RB, Lynch J, McCulloch CE, Majumdar S, Lane NE, Link TM. Scoring hip osteoarthritis with MRI (SHOMRI): a whole joint oste-oarthritis evaluation system. J Magn Reson Imaging 2015;41(6):1549−57.

[20] Noble CA. The treatment of iliotibial band friction syndrome. Br J Sports Med 1979;13: 51−4.

[21] Souza RB, Powers CM. Concurrent criterion-related validity and reliability of a clinical test to measure femoral anteversion. J Orthop Sports Phys Ther 2009;39(8):586−92.

[22] Groh MM, Herrera J. A comprehensive review of hip labral tears. Curr Rev Musculos-kelet Med 2009;2(2):105−17.

[23] Johnson AW, Weiss Jr CB, Wheeler DL. Stress fractures of the femoral shaft in athletes− more common than expected. A new clinical test. Am J Sports Med 1994;22(2): 248−56.

[24] Cuckler JM. Limb length and stability in total hip replacement. Orthopedics 2005; 28(9):951−3.

[25] Doherty M, Courtney P, Doherty S, Jenkins W, Maciewicz RA, Muir K, Zhang W. Nonspherical femoral head shape (pistol grip deformity), neck shaft angle, and risk of hip osteoarthritis: a case-control study. Arthritis Rheum 2008;58(10):3172–82.

[26] Miao M, Cai H, Hu L, Wang Z. Retrospective observational study comparing the international hip dysplasia institute classification with the Tonnisclassification of developmental dysplasia of the hip. Medicine 2017;96(3):e5902.

[27] Milasinovic S, Brdar R, Petronic I, Nikolic D, Cirovic D. Developmental dysplasia of the hip - angle trends after operation in different age groups. Arch Med Sci 2010;6(5):800–5.

[28] Apley AG, Wientroub S. The sagging rope sign in Perthes' disease and allied disorders. J Bone Jt Surg Br 1981;63-B(1):43–7.

[29] Loder RT, Aronsson DD, Weinstein SL, Breur GJ, Ganz R, Leunig M. Slipped capital femoral epiphysis. Instr Course Lect 2008;57:473–98.

Deformities

Coxa valga

Increase in neck shaft angle in the frontal plane (angle of inclination >125 degrees) in adults is known as coxavalga [1]. Normally, the angle of inclination in newborn is about 150 degrees which gradually decreases to 120 degrees as the child stand, walk, and bear wt. Persistent increase in neck shaft angle is known as coxavalga, which is often associated with femoral anteversion. Coxavalga is associated with shallow acetabulum and associated anteversion make the joint relatively unstable.

Unilateral coxavalga increases the supratrochanteric height of femur and leg length discrepancy. In case of LLD, one may stand by bending the hip and knee on the affected side bearing more load on the opposite limb or stands by plantar flexion of opposite ankle joint bearing more load on the affected limb. While walking, the affected longer limb bears more load during loading phase of each gait cycle as the weight line shifts away from affected hip joint increasing the weight-arm.

In coxavalga, the effort arm is reduced. So, the Trendelenburg sign become positive and walks with painless lurching on the affected side. Increased load bearing on the head of affected femur during loading phase of each gait cycle may lead to early degeneration over time.

There will be pelvic tilt with adduction of the affected hip and overtime, one may develop hip adductor shortening. Hip adduction leads to further instability of the hip jt. There will be compensatory bending of L-spine toward the affected side. One may develop scoliosis with the convexity toward the sound side. Pelvic tilt and unequal weight bearing may predispose to sacroiliac joint stress and strain. Scoliosis may result in LBP.

In coxa valga, the bending moment arm across the femoral neck is reduced [2]. This situation also decreases the vertical shear across the femoral neck. The valgus position may also increase the functional length of the hip abductor muscles, thus improving their force-generating ability.

The negative effect of coxa valga is the decreased moment arm available to the hip abductor force. In extreme coxa valga, the femoral head may be positioned more laterally in the acetabulum, possibly increasing the risk of dislocation.

Causes—Lack of weight bearing due to Ceberal Palsy, any other neurological disorders that delay the weight bearing may result in persistent increase in neck shaft angle [3].

Clinical Feature—One walks with painless limping on the affected side and stand either flexing the affected hip and knee bearing more loads on the sound side and/or plantar flexion of the opposite foot bearing more loads on the affected hip.

Inspection
- Pelvic tilt present with the affected side up.
- Hip abduction range on the affected side may be more in early ages, which may decrease over time due to adaptive shortening of hip adductors.
- Hip internal rotation range may be greater than external rotation suggestive of associated anteversion.
- Trendelenburg sign is positive.

Special test
- GT lies below the Nelaton's line
- Schoemaker's line bisect the midline above the umbilicus
- Bryant's triangle shows supratrochanteric length of femur is increased.

Treatment
- Since it is a bony deformity, not expected to be corrected by therapy. To equalize the limb length so that both the extremities will bear almost equal load during standing as well as walking, foot wear compensation with the heel and sole raise may be given on the opposite side.
- Hip abductor strengthening of the affected side and stretching of hip adductors. In a growing child, on weight bearing, the coxavalga may reduce over time.
- In case of severe coxavalga, corrective osteotomy is indicated. Medial close wedge osteotomy is done. To correct the anteversion, derotation is performed and the fragments are fixed by internal fixation followed by immobilization [4].

Coxa vara

Reduced neck shaft angle <120 degrees is known as coxavara.

The change in the angle causes mechanical restriction of abduction at hip, shortening of the limb and waddling gait [5].

Causes
1. Congenital (Infantile)—It is usually bilateral and may present with pain and stiffness of the hip. It is characterized by a triangular defect in the inferior

portion of the neck of the femur(in AP view X-ray) [6]. On examination, the GT is overridden with resultant shortening of the limb, limitation of the rotation, and abduction of the limb.

2. Developmental—Most are not diagnosed at birth but rather present when the child begins to ambulate with a Trendelenburg limp. The pathognomic radiologic sign is the inferior and posterior bony metaphyseal fragment in the femoral neck.

3. Dysplastic—Due to an underlying bony abnormality such as fibrous dysplasia, Vitamin D deficiency, rickets, osteoporosis and various generalized skeletal dysplasia (spondylometaphyseal, spondyloepiphyseal, and cleidocranial dysplasias).

4. Epiphyseal (slipped capital femoral epiphysis)—It is very common in adolescent male. Sudden or gradual slip of the upper femoral epiphysis resulting in coxavara due to strain on the growing epiphysis, cause may be trauma or imbalance between growth and sex hormones [7]. Abduction, internal rotation, hyperextension is restricted. Characteristic sign is external rotation of the hip when hip and knee are flexed.

5. Deformity that causes a decreased joint load because of more balanced force distribution. The femoral neck tends to be shorter. The head maintains a more central position in the acetabulum because of the greater leverage associated with the adductors. This deformity, however, causes more shearing forces that can lead to a pseudoarthrosis of the femoral neck.

6. Fracture neck of femur, fracture trochanter, usually heals with coxavara.

7. Rickets—Weight bearing increases the bending movement and result in coxavara.

Unilateral coxavara is associated with supratrochanteric shortening of neck of femur and LLD on the affected side [8]. Since the bending moment is increased, there is increased chance of fracture neck of femur. As the GT approximates the bone of origin of the hip abductors, the hip abductors remain in mechanically disadvantageous position as per the length tension relationship. So, the Trendelenburg sign will be positive. Patient stands with hip-knee flexion on the opposite side bearing more loads on the affected side or with plantar flexion on the affected side ankle bearing more loads on the sound side and walks with painless lurching on the affected side.

Since there is LLD with affected side shortening patient walks bearing more loads on the sound side. During loading phase of each gait cycle, sound side hip tends to be adducted and overtime hip abduction range will be limited due to adaptive shortening of hip abductors. Affected side hip abduction range may be limited due to premature bony contact with the GT. It may associate with femoral retroversion. Pelvic tilt give rise to scoliosis and one may develop LBP.

The varus position increases the moment arm of the hip abductor force [9]. The greater leverage increases the abduction torque produced per unit of hip abductor muscle force. This situation may benefit people with hip abductor weakness.

Increasing the leverage of the abductor muscles may allow a given level of abduction torque required during the stance phase of walking to be generated by less muscle force. Such reduction of muscular-based joint forces can help protect an arthritic or unstable prosthetic hip from excessive wear during walking.

A varus osteotomy may in some patients improve the stability of the joint by aligning the femoral head more directly into the acetabulum.

A potentially negative effect of coxa vara is an increased bending moment (or torque) generated across the femoral neck. The bending moment arm increases as the angle of inclination approaches 90 degrees. Increasing the bending moment raises the tension across the superior aspect of the femoral neck. This situation may cause a fracture of the femoral neck or a structural failure of a prosthesis. Marked coxa vara increases the vertical shear between the femoral head and the adjacent epiphysis. In children, this situation may lead to a condition known as a slipped capital femoral epiphysis. Coxa vara may also decrease the functional length of the hip abductor muscles, thereby reducing the force-generating capability of these muscles and increasing the likelihood of a "gluteus medius limp." [10] The loss in muscle force may offset the increased abduction torque potential gained by the increased hip abductor moment arm.

Clinical Feature—Patient walks with painless limping on the affected side. On inspection, one may stand with plantar flexion of the affected side or hip knee flexion of opposite side. Pelvic tilt and scoliosis may be present.

Movements—Affected side hip abduction range limited with bony block. Increases in hip external rotation range suggest associated retroversion. Unaffected side hip abduction range may be limited due to adaptive shortening of hip adductors.

Special tests

- GT lies above the Nelaton's line.
- Bryant's triangle shows supratrochanteric shortening
- Schoemaker's line bisect the midline below the umbilicus
- Trendelenburg sign positive.
- True LLD as well as apparent LLD present due to supratrochanteric shortening.
- The sound side head of femur bears more load during each loading phase of gait cycle due to LLD. Overtime, it undergoes degeneration and secondary OA of the hip jt.

Management—Footwear compensation on affected side to equalize the limb length, so that bilateral symmetrical load bearing is promoted. Progressive resisted exercises for the hip abductors, stretching of adductors on the sound side. In severe case, medical open wedge intertrochanteric osteotomy with bone graft and internal fixation may be performed.

Anteversion

Persistent increase in neck shaft angle in transverse plane more than 15 degrees is referred as anteversion. There is internal rotation around the long axis of the femur.

Anteversion is characterized by increased hip internal rotation range at the cost of external rotation. It is often associated with coxavalga [11].

It is important to note that internal rotation of the hip is not the same as internal torsion of the femur. Femoral torsion is rotation within a bone itself, a twisting of the bone, whereas internal rotation of the hip occurs between bones, at the coxa-femoral joint. It results in a change in the orientation of the femoral condyles in the transverse plane. So, observing the client's knees anteriorly and posteriorly can be helpful in identifying internal rotation of the hip. With both internal rotation of the hip and internal femoral torsion, the lateral femoral condyle is orientated more anteriorly than normal and the medial femoral condyle is orientated more posteriorly.

A patient with this posture may have a characteristic toe-in foot position, where the tibia is also internally rotated, or the foot position may be neutral. Whether the foot position is toe-in or neutral, the patella faces inward, which is one way to identify this posture. However, unlike some of the other postures with signs that are visibly apparent, the degree of inward rotation of the femur is more difficult to identify from postural assessment alone, and for this reason muscle length tests are important for determining whether a patient has a reduction in external hip rotation, which is a corresponding finding with this posture.

Consequences of internal rotation of the hip

With increased internal hip rotation, there is corresponding decreased external rotation in the coxa-femoral joint. Internal rotators are shortened and external rotators are lengthened. Both muscle groups may be weakened because they are not functioning at their optimal length or within their optimal range. Weakness in external rotators of the hip is associated with musculoskeletal disorders of the knee such as patellofemoral joint pain syndrome and noncontact injury to the anterior cruciate ligament in adolescent girls [12]. Imbalance in muscles around the hip joint could affect function of the joint and ultimately affect not only gait but also functional and sporting activities. Femoral torsion can be a contributing factor to internal rotation of the hip. The degree of femoral torsion is described as an angle that is formed by a line drawn longitudinally through the neck of the femur superimposed over a line drawn between the femoral condyles. This angle is usually 10–15 degrees but varies widely. An increase in torsion angle is called anteversion. Anteversion can cause compensatory change in the hip joint and affect weight bearing, muscle biomechanics and hip joint stability and may also create dysfunction at the knee and foot. Internal rotation of the hip changes the normal orientation of the femoral head within the acetabulum. Prolonged alteration in the distribution of forces through the articular surfaces of the hip joint could predispose the joint to degenerative changes in the bone, articular cartilage and connective tissue. Internal rotation of the hip threatens to pinch anterior hip structures, causing pain. With internal rotation of the femur, there is abnormal orientation of the knee joint. This is exacerbated where there is a neutral foot position because this requires external rotation of the tibia in cases where internal rotation of the femur is present. Altered hip and knee biomechanics alter both walking and running ability and could therefore adversely affect participation in recreational and sporting activities. Where internal rotation is due to torsional deformity of the femur, this could contribute to arthritis in the knee joint: internal femoral torsion increases pressure on the lateral facet, producing anterior knee pain and patellofemoral arthritis [13]. There may be lateral patellar subluxation. Internal rotation of the hip is often accompanied by subtalar pronation of the foot, and this too causes problems (Fig. 3.1).

One stands and walks with in toeing gait. In standing, both the patella faces inward known as squinting patella proportionately more anterior portion of head of femur remains uncovered by the acetabular cavity resulting in instability. There is increased Q angle and genu valgum. The patella tracks laterally by the resultant of quadriceps force system in the frontal plane, which is referred as lateral tracking dysfunction of patella. It may give rise to anterior knee pain.

Anteversion is associated with pronated foot [14]. On weight bearing, the plantar capsulo-ligamentous structures are stretched, so one complains of foot pain. The pain disappears after sometimes due to protective contraction of the muscles and returns back with increased intensity due to fatigue.

Pronated foot and genu valgum results in shortening of the extremity, infrapelvic tilt, and scoliosis. To cover the anterior part of head of femur, there may occur compensatory anterior pelvic tilt. scoliosis and increased lumbar lordosis may give rise to LBP.

One may develop compensatory external tibial torsion, which is characterized by squinting patella with normal foot orientation.

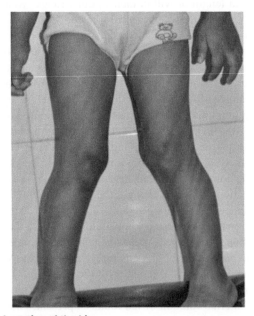

FIGURE 3.1 Internal rotation of the hip.

Management

Acknowledge that where internal rotation is the result of bony anatomy, such as femoral torsion. Nonsurgical intervention to correct internal hip rotation is limited. Apply passive stretches to internal rotators. Stretching tensor fasciae latae may be particularly important in the treatment of internal hip rotation.

Use soft tissue release to lengthen gluteus medius. With the hip in a neutral position, gently lock the muscle using your thumb or elbow and then use your other hand to move your client's leg (as if testing for external rotation) while maintaining the lock. Massage and passively stretch adductors on the affected side. Use MFR longitudinal leg pulls because these can relax all muscles of the hip joint and the entire lower limb before using some of the previously described techniques.

Discourage the child W-sitting position (Internal rotation of femur + genu valgum, leads to anteversion) and encourage cross-sitting. External rotation of the hip in supine position and knee straight should be encouraged. Progressive strengthening of hip external rotators should be given. In case of unilateral anteversion, foot wear modification with medial heel and sole raise, and medial arch support and if require, compensation may be given. In case of severe deformity, derotational osteotomy may be considered.

Retroversion

Reduced neck shaft angle less than 15 degrees in transverse plane is known as retroversion. It is characterized by out-toeing gait (Fig. 3.2). Hip external rotation range is increased at the cost of internal rotation.

Retroversion is associated with genu varum and supination of the foot [15]. The Q angle will be reduced. Increased vertical compressive load on the medial compartment of tibio-femoral joint predispose to DJD. One may develop compensatory reduced external tibial torsion during the growing age. Foot supination results in increased medial longitudinal arch, rigid foot, increased leg length, pelvic tilt, reduced shock absorption may lead to foot pain. Unilateral retroversion with supination of foot may result in LLD (affected side longer) pelvic tilt, scoliosis, and LBP. Shifting of line of gravity away from affected side loads the affected hip to a greater extent during mid-stance phase of each gait cycle predisposing to degeneration.

Management—In a growing child facilitates the position of hip internal rotation, that is, W sitting. Stretching of hip external rotator and strengthening of hip internal rotators should be encouraged. In case of severe deformity, derotational osteotomy may be considered.

Hip flexion deformity

Hip flexion deformity is very common acquired deformity in hip joint. Hip flexion being the resting position, in case of any hip pathology one assumes hip flexion for position for comfort. Over time hip flexion deformity due to adoptive shortening of

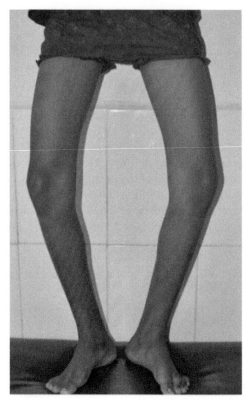

FIGURE 3.2 Retroversion of hip.

hip flexors develops. In any types of arthritis, spasm of hip flexors and adductors often develop in acute stage. In case of postpolio residual paralysis, spina bifida, muscular dystrophy, etc. neuro-muscular conditions hip flexion deformity develops due to muscle imbalance. It is often associated with knee flexion deformity and vice versa [16].

Hip flexion deformity is always transformed to its bone of origin, pelvis, and lumbar spine. One with hip flexion deformity lies down in supine lying position with the thigh touching the bed. However, lumbar lordosis is exaggerated. Once the lordosis is flattened by flexing the sound hip, the original hip flexion deformity appears and can be measured by the goniometer.

In case of hip flexion deformity, one stands and walks with increased lumbar lordosis. Normally hip joint is in neutral position, which is the closed crack and most congruent position of the joint, at each midstance phase of gait cycle. Loading the hip in closed pack position reduces the load on it. In case of hip flexion defor-mity, the joint is loaded in semiflexed position, which is incongruent. So, the load over it increases at each midstance phase of gait cycle. Over time it undergoes degeneration. Hip flexion deformity is one of the predisposing factors for early osteoarthritis. Associated increase lumbar lordosis may results in low back pain. There will be shortening of the affected side and to compensate it one stands with ankle plantar flexion.

Pelvic tilt
Anterior pelvic tilt

Normally both ASIS are leveled when viewed from the front with the patient in standing posture and both PSIS are also leveled when viewed from behind. Side views from both the sides ASIS levels with PSIS. Normally, ASIS & symphysis pubis lies on frontal or coronal plane. Deviation from the normal alignment is known as pelvic tilt.

In case of anterior pelvic tilt both ASIS are lower than both the PSIS as viewed from both the sides. The lumbar lordosis gets exaggerated that is hyper extension of lumbar spine occurs [17].

Abdominals and hip extensors form a forced couple that tilts the pelvis backward and back extensor and hip flexor forms another forced couple that tilts the pelvis forward. These four groups of muscles are attached to the pelvis or lumbar spine. Balance between the two force couples results in normal lumbo-pelvic posture. Imbalance between the two may lead to pelvic tilt. Tightness of the hip flexors, weakness of the abdominals, over stretching/shortening of back extensors weakness of hip extensor may produce anterior pelvic tilt. Anterior pelvic tilt also develops in case of obesity, pregnancy, protruded abdomen due to intraabdominal mass or swelling. In case of protruded abdomen center of gravity shifts forward and to bring the line of gravity over base of support, one leans/bends backward from the L-Spine.

In case of anterior pelvic tilt and increased lumbar lordosis, there occurs compression on the posterior elements of the spine and distraction on the anterior part. Increase compressive force over posterior elements may lead to failure of the pars interarticularis as the posterior located facet joint can bear maximum about one-third of the body weight. Failure of pars interarticularis results in fracture, which is referred as **Spondylosis** [18]. In case of lumbo-sacral instability due to Spondylosis, degeneration, hyperextension of L-spine predisposes to posterior to anterior slippage of the vertebrae with the vertebral column above it as extension of spine is associated with posterior to anterior translation of vertebrae. Hyperextension of L-spine reduces the size of IVF referred as **foraminal stenosis** that may compress its content like spinal nerve root, giving rise to radicular pain. Increase vertical compressive load over the facet joint leads to progressive degeneration of the articular cartilage and facet joint arthropathy. Increase in vertical compressive load over the posterior annulus fibrosus leads to thinning of posterior annulus fibrosus. It may fail to withstand increase vertical compressive load and degenerate over time.

Cleft develops in posterior annulus fibrosus and it ruptures as it fails to withstand the horizontal stress exerted by the nucleus pulposus. This gives rise to posterior derangement/herniated disc lesion/PIVD. Over time there may develop adaptive shortening of posterior vertebral soft tissue structure resulting in flexion dysfunction. Increase in lumbar lordosis is often associated with hip flexion deformity. Usually LOG shifts behind the lumbo-spinal hip joint and anterior to the knee joint. Substitution of hip, lumbar extensors, and knee extensors by the gravity may result in weakness of these groups of muscles. It may be associated with increase kyphosis and head forward posture.

Management—To restore the normal lumbo-pelvic alignments, find out the underlying cause. Hip flexor stretching, strengthening of abdominals are mostly required [19]. One may require stretching of the T-L fascia and the back extensors, posterior soft tissue structures and strengthening of gluteus maximus. For lumbar flexion, caudal to cephalic, flexion can be given in supine lying position. Flexion with knee straight is more effective than that with hips and knees flexed. In lumbar flexion, cephal to caudal movement can be given in supine lying with the clasp of finger behind the neck and bend elbows are the fulcrum. Lumbar flexion can also be given in high sitting position by applying pressure from the shoulder as per the bending principle. William's flexion exercise, McKenzie lumbar flexion is also useful. Patient can be advised to do rocking movement lying in trunk prone lying position with a pillow under the abdomen.

Posterior pelvic tilt

It is characterized by both the PSISs lying downward as compared to both the ASISs as viewed from both the sides. Lumbar lordosis is reduced, flattened, or reversed. Posterior pelvic tilt occurs due to shortening of the hamstrings weakness of back extensors [20]. Posterior pelvic tilt may occur as a compensatory mechanism to various painful conditions such as PIVD, AS, etc.

Normal lumbar lordotic posture is considered as close pack position which is the most stable posture. Reduce lumbar lordosis/flattening is unstable lumbar posture which requires more muscle activity to maintain the posture. The compression-distraction effect on spine depends on the extent of posterior pelvic tilt. In case of flattening of the L-spine there may be equal anterior—posterior compression-distraction, where as in case of kyphotic L-spine there will be more anterior compression and posterior distraction. Anterior compression shifts the gel like nucleus pulposus backwards predisposing to PIVD. The vertical compressive load gets transmitted to the anterior element, that is, IV joints and deloads the posteriorly located facet joints. Compression of the facet joint may predispose to degeneration of the articular cartilage.

Management—To restore the normal Lumbar lordosis which is the stable posture is the aim of management. Depending on the underlying cause the treatment may be planned. Stretching of the hamstrings, McKenzie repeated extension exercise; back extensors strengthening, etc. are used. One may require Maitland's rhythmic central PA mobilization over spinous processes. Bilateral pressure on articular pillar to restore the lordosis. Use of lumbar roll during sitting and lying is recommended.

Infrapelvic tilt

Pelvic tilt in coronal plane may occur in downward direction or upward direction. Infrapelvic tilt is usually due to hip abductor shortening. It may also occur to compensate LLD on the shorter side. Suprapelvic tilt occurs in case of hip adductor shortening, in spastic hemi-paresis, persistent ATNR [21]. Suprapelvic tilt may occur on the longer side to compensate LLD.

In case of hip abductor shortening, one bends the trunk forward to the affected side to place the abducted hip in contact with the ground. Both the lower limbs appear parallel to each other; however, hip abduction deformity is compensated by infrapelvic tilt.

In case of infrapelvic tilt, affected hip is abducted and opposite hip is adducted. There may develop apparent LLD, that is, affected side appear longer so one may stand either with PF of the opposite foot bearing more weight on affected side or knee flexion of the affected side and bears more weight on the sound side. During walking, LOG shifts toward the affected side. Thus, the weight arm from the hip joint axis is reduced. So, the hip abductor muscle force on affected side balance the pelvis is also proportionately decreased, that is, the net loading during the mid-stance phase on the affected hip is reduced whereas that on the opposite side will be increased. It predisposes the opposite hip to secondary degeneration.

One may stand with the affected hip in abduction. It leads to genu valgum and foot pronation (flat foot) [22]. If one stands with equinus foot on the opposite side bearing almost all the weight on the affected he is likely to develop pain on the weight bearing joints of the affected extremity. Some other compensate by flexing the affected hip and knee, weight bearing on the sound limb during standing may give rise to pain on the sound side weight bearing joints.

The hip which is abducted is relatively most stable than the hip which is adducted, that is, opposite side hip is liable to develop subluxation. Pelvic tilt is compensated with scoliosis with the convexity toward affected side and may develop unequal weight bearing may predispose to SI stress and LBP.

Management—It depends on the cause. Stretching of hip abductors is required. Find out the underlying cause for the hip abduction shortening. It may develop due to muscle imbalance, which requires adductor strengthening. Hip flexion-abduction and knee flexion often occur due to adaptive positioning to get relief from any painful hip or knee condition. Unless the painful arthritis is treated hip abductor tightness and pelvic t/t cannot be corrected. To accommodate the deformity foot wear compensation to the opposite side may be given, so that one can bear almost equal weight when standing.

Suprapelvic tilt

Suprapelvic tilt occurs in case of hip adductor shortening, spastic hemi paresis, persistent ATNR. Suprapelvic tilt may occur in the longer side to compensate

LLD. Maybe associated with scoliosis that affect the breathing [1]. One may stand by equinus foot on the affected side/knee flexion on the sound side or hip abduction on the sound side. To stand with both the foot flat on the ground and almost equal weight bearing on both the legs, foot wear compensation on the affected side may be given. While walking LOG shifts toward the opposite hip thus, affected side hip bears more weight during midstance phase of each GAIT cycle predisposing to degenerative arthritis. Associated scoliosis may affect the breathing. Unequal weight bearing may predispose to SI joint compression and pain.

Management—Stretching of hip adductor, footwear compensation on the involved side, deep breathing exercises, rocking exercise to correct the scoliosis may be performed.

References

[1] Isaac B, Vettivel S, Prasad R, Jeyaseelan L, Chandi G. Prediction of the femoral neck-shaft angle from the length of the femoral neck. Clin Anat 1997;10(5):318−23.

[2] Harris JD, Chahal J. Femoral neck stress fractures. Open Tech Sports Med 2015;23(3): 241−7.

[3] Morrell DS, Pearson M, Sauser DD. Progressive bone and joint abnormalities of the spine and lower extremities in cerebral Palsy. Radiographics 2002;22(2):257−68.

[4] Moens P, Lammens J, Molenaers G, Fabry G. Femoral derotation for increased hip anteversion. A new surgical technique with a modified Ilizarov frame. J Bone Jt Surg Br 1995;77(1):107−9.

[5] Mazzini JP, Martín JR, Ciruelos RM. Coxa vara with proximal femoral growth arrest as a possible consequence of extracorporeal membrane oxygenation: a case report. Cases J 2009;2:8130.

[6] Kim HT, Chambers HG, Mubarak SJ, Wenger DR. Congenital coxa vara: computed tomographic analysis of femoral retroversion and the triangular metaphyseal fragment. J Pediatr Orthop 2000;20(5):551−6.

[7] Key JA. The classic: epiphyseal coxa vara or displacement of the capital epiphysis of the femur in adolescence. Clin Orthop Relat Res 2013;471(7):2087−117.

[8] QorrajBytyqi H, Bytyqi C. Management of coxa vara septica and pseudoarthrosis of the femoral neck: a case report. Am J Case Rep 2017;18:440−3.

[9] Henderson E, Marulanda G, Cheong D, Temple H, Letson G. Hip abductor moment arm - a mathematical analysis for proximal femoral replacement. J Orthop Surg Res 2011; 6(1):6.

[10] Lung K, Lui F. Anatomy, abdomen and pelvis, superior gluteal nerve [Updated 2021 Aug 11]. In: StatPearls [Internet]. Treasure Island (FL): StatPearls Publishing; 2022. https://www.ncbi.nlm.nih.gov/books/NBK535408/.

[11] Buly RL. Femoral deformities: valgus, varus, retroversion, and anteversion. In: Nho S, Leunig M, Kelly B, Bedi A, Larson C, editors. Hip arthroscopy and hip joint preservation surgery. New York, NY: Springer; 2014. https://doi.org/10.1007/978-1-4614-7321-3_52-1.

[12] Powers CM. The influence of abnormal hip mechanics on knee injury: a biomechanical perspective. J Orthop Sports Phys Ther 2010;40(2):42−51.

[13] Snow M. Tibial torsion and patellofemoral pain and instability in the adult population: current concept review. Curr Rev Musculoskelet Med 2021;14(1):67–75.

[14] Gandhi N, Salvi R. Correlation between pronated foot and pelvic inclination, femoral anteversion, quadriceps angle and tibial torsion. Int J Physiother 2017;4(4).

[15] Khamis S, Dar G, Peretz C, Yizhar Z. The relationship between foot and pelvic alignment while standing. J Hum Kinet 2015;46:85–97.

[16] Kellis E, Ellinoudis A, Kofotolis N. Effect of hip flexion angle on the hamstring to quadriceps strength ratio. Sports 2019;7(2):43.

[17] Levine D, Whittle MW. The effects of pelvic movement on lumbar lordosis in the standing position. J Orthop Sports Phys Ther 1996;24(3):130–5.

[18] Pereira Duarte M, Camino Willhuber GO. Pars interarticularis injury [Updated 2021 Aug 11]. In: StatPearls [Internet]. Treasure Island (FL): StatPearls Publishing; 2022. https://www.ncbi.nlm.nih.gov/books/NBK545191/.

[19] Avrahami D, Potvin JR. The clinical and biomechanical effects of fascial-muscular lengthening therapy on tight hip flexor patients with and without low back pain. J Can Chiropr Assoc 2014;58(4):444–55.

[20] Jandre Reis FJ, Macedo AR. Influence of hamstring tightness in pelvic, lumbar and trunk range of motion in low back pain and asymptomatic volunteers during forward bending. Asian Spine J 2015;9(4):535–40.

[21] Husson JL, Mallet JF, Huten D, Odri GA, Morin C, Parent HF. The lumbar-pelvic-femoral complex: applications in hip pathology. J Orthop Traumatol: Surgery & Research 2010;96(4):S10–6.

[22] Khamis S, Yizhar Z. Effect of feet hyperpronation on pelvic alignment in a standing position. Gait Posture 2007;25(1):127–34.

Further reading

[1] Koumbourlis AC. Scoliosis and the respiratory system. Paediatr Respir Rev 2006;7(2): 152–60.

Arthritis conditions

Osteoarthritis/degenerative joint disease of hip joint

It is the progressive degeneration of articular cartilage with compensatory collagenous and bony proliferation [1]. The incidence of OA hip is relatively less in Indian population as compared to OA knee [2]. Incidence of OA hip is more in western population whereas incidence of OA knee is more common in Indian population probably due to nature of activities of daily living.

Causes

The exact cause is not known. There are various hypothesis regarding the cause of OA Hip:

1. **Aging**—As OA hip occurs in elderly population, it is thought to be due to aging. If it would have been due to aging, nonarticulating portion of articular cartilage would have been degenerated but in OA hip, the articulating portion of articular cartilage undergo degeneration. So, the aging theory is rejected. The avascular articular cartilage derives its nutrition from synovial fluid by the process of diffusion. It requires alternate compression and relaxation of articular cartilage to get fresh nutrition. During compression, the used synovial fluid with metabolic waste product is squeezed out of articular cartilage and during relaxation, articular cartilage receives fresh synovial fluid and nutrition. Since the nonarticular portion of articular cartilage lacks compression and relaxation, it devoids of nutrition and is supposed to undergo degeneration [3]. In OA hip, as the articular portion of articular cartilage undergoes degeneration, the aging theory is rejected.
2. **Wear and tear theory**—It is a continuous process. Normally, the rate of tissue damage is equal to rate of tissue repair. Since articular cartilage is a smooth frictionless surface, this theory is not acceptable [4].
3. **Loading**—More is the loading, more is the articular cartilage damage, but, not all obese/overweight individuals develop Osteoarthritis. Whereas persons with low body weight/thin individual often develop OA hip, so the loading theory is also not acceptable. An experiment was performed, by subjecting Rabbit's knee to load equal to the body weight at the rate of 60/min, 1 h daily

Physiotherapy for the Hip Joint. https://doi.org/10.1016/B978-0-323-93649-1.00011-9

for 1month. It has been found that gross OA changes was in Rabbit's knee after 1 month. It was concluded that it is not the magnitude of the load, it is the nature of the load that is responsible for degeneration. An obese person performs weight bearing activities in congruent/near congruent position of hip joint may not develop degeneration, whereas a thin individual, if performs weight bearing activities in incongruent position it likely to develop degeneration [5].

4. **Elasticity of tissue**—Energy attenuation capacity of any tissue is directly proportional to its elasticity. More elastic is the articular cartilage, it absorbs more load and less load will be transferred to the underlying subchondral bone. Less elastic is the articular cartilage bone due to hardening/sclerosis, more load acts over the subchondral bone that may cause degeneration [6].

5. **Periarticular muscle strength**—Eccentric work of muscle is an excellent means to protect the joint. Stronger muscles deload the joint and protect the articular cartilage. Weaker is the muscle around the joint, more is the joint loading and more is the chance of degeneration.

6. **Leg-length discrepancy**—In case of LLD, one bends the longer side hip and knee and bears more load on the shorter side and/or plantar flexing the shorter side ankle to bear more load on the longer side during standing [7]. During walking, the shorter side bears less load during loading phase of each gait cycle. The LOG shifts toward the shorter side, increasing the weight arm on the longer side, so the longer side bears more loads during loading phase of each gait cycle. So, the longer side is likely to develop progressive degeneration.

7. **Hip flexion deformity**—Normally, the hip joint is loaded in neutral extension at mid-stance phase of each gait cycle which is the congruent position, so joint loading is the least (Load = Force per unit area, the area of contact is increased here). In case of hip flexion deformity, the hip joint fails to attain the closed packed position. Loading in flexion which is incongruent increases the load and predispose to degeneration.

8. **Increased body weight**—1 kg increased in body weight adds 3 kg to the hip jt during midstance phase of each gait cycle. So, obesity/overweight may be one of the predisposing factors.

9. **Genetics**—Since, the incidence of OA is more common in familial involvement as it is genetic.

Primary OA can be differentiated from secondary by the elimination of preexisting/precipitating factors such as injury, fracture, dislocation, coxavalga, coxavara, AVN of head of femur, RA, septic Arthritis, LLD, etc.

Pathology

The degeneration starts from the area of articular cartilage subjected to greater compressive load. It starts with the loss of mucopolysaccharide and proportionate loss of water content. With the loss of water content the energy attenuation capacity of articular cartilage is impaired, now the cells will be subjected to greater load. There occurs cell death [8]. The dead portion of articular cartilage gets detached from parent body and fissure develops. To remove the necrosed articular cartilage out of joint cavity, there develop synovitis. Gradually, the synovitis resolves and healing occur by compensatory collagenous and bony proliferation as the avascular articular cartilage cannot be repaired/replaced. With the resolution of synovitis, capsular fibrosis and limitation of JROM in capsular pattern develops. Pain due to synovitis inhibits the muscle, disuse atrophy, and muscle weakness develops. Gradually progressive degeneration of articular cartilage may involve the subchondral bone, joint become laxed, and unstable. Involvement of highly neural subchondral bone gives rise to continuous pain.

- **Fibrillation stage** is characterized by pain following activities due to fatigue.
- **Fissure**—detachment of necrosed articular cartilage and synovitis give rise to chemical pain.
- Compensatory capsular fibrosis limits the movement in capsular pattern and the movement/activities that stretches the tight joint capsule cause pain.
- Involvement of subchondral bone causes continuous pain and joint instability that requires joint replacement and arthroplasty.

Clinical features

Patients complain of insidious onset of pain in the hip joint following activities, due to fatigue. The period of pain-free state gradually reduces. With the onset of inflammation, one complains of morning pain and stiffness that reduces with movement and activities and returns back with increased intensity following activities. Gradually, movement gets restricted in capsular pattern and one complains of pain during movement and activities that stretches the tight joint capsule. One may experience pain during walking as tight anterior joint capsule stretches following midstance phase of gait cycle. Crossed legged sitting, squatting may be painful due to shortening of posterolateral joint capsule.

One walks with limping on the affected side. Wasting of the gluteus may be present. Shortening (supratrochanteric) may be present with infrapelvic tilt.

Movement evaluation

Weight bearing, single leg standing, Trendelenburg sign may be positive. Squatting, cross leg sitting may be limited and painful. Active nonweight bearing physiological movement is limited in capsular pattern, that is, hip extension, internal rotation, and abduction will be limited. Crepitus may be present. Resisted isometric hip extension, abduction may be weak.

On palpation glutei wasting may be present.

Management

Degenerative joint diseases (DJD) involve the aneural articular cartilage, so one is not supposed to feel the pain. The source of pain in DJD in the initial stage could be due to fatigue, that is, the reason why one feels the pain following activities. Later on, as inflammation set in, inflammatory exudates irritate/compress the nerve ending present in the joint capsule and give rise to pain. In the third stage, joint capsule give rise to pain. In the third stage, joint hypomobility due to capsular tightness produces pain as the short joint capsule gets stretched and in the fourth stage, involvement of highly neural subchondral bone produces almost continuous pain. There is hypomobility and crepitus present [9].

Since, articular cartilage is avascular structure, having poor metabolic capacity, it cannot be repaired/replaced so protection of joint to prevent/minimize progression of degeneration is the aim of management.

Minimize the weight bearing activities. One should avoid standing and walking as much as possible. While standing, stand with one leg forward or over a height (step) with one hand support and keep on changing leg position. Use ramp and elevator instead of steps. Stretch hip flexors and piriformis so that during walking weight bearing in congruent position could be possible, thus reducing joint loading. Strengthening of glutei by isometric gluteus maximus, theraband hip abductor exercise should be encouraged. Stretching of bilateral hip adductors in standing with hand support should be practiced in morning and evening.

In the synovitis stage (acute), antiinflammatory drug therapy is mandatory and physiotherapy has little role. One can practice isometric gluteal exercise, nonweight bearing hip movement, IFT, HVPGS, strong faradic stimulation to glutei, LASER can be used to resolve the inflammation, relieve the pain, facilitates muscle contraction.

During the hypomobile stage, physiotherapy aims to restore full range of joint movement by mobilization technique and passive stretching. Cyriax's forced extension, internal rotation to stretch the anterior and posterior joint capsule, respectively, can be used.

As per Maitland's concept anterior to posterior glide to improve flexion and internal rotation ROM can be used. A-P glide through long axis of femur with hip flexed to 90 and knee in full flexion is more useful. Scouring is an effective means to stretch posterolateral joint capsule to improve internal rotation and flexion. For extension, PA glide can be used. As per Mulligan technique, mobilization with movement in nonweight bearing or weight bearing can be given to restore pain free full ROM. In the fourth stage, when subchondral bone is involved, replacement arthroplasty is indicated. One should use walking stick on opposite side to deload the joint. Use railing while walking or climbing the stairs.

Rheumatoid arthritis (RA)

Rheumatoid arthritis (RA) is a chronic autoimmune disease that causes severe pain, stiffness, and swelling in the lining of the joints. RA can affect different parts of the body, including bilateral symmetrical joints involvement in the hands, feet, and knees. But RA can affect any joint, including the hip joint and shoulders. About 15%–28% of people with RA develop hip RA. Most people with hip RA experience it later on as their RA progresses. RA is a chronic inflammatory disorder that can affect wide variety of body systems other than joints including the skin, eyes, lungs, heart, and blood vessels.

Epidemiology

Worldwide, the annual incidence of RA is approximately 3 cases per 10,000 population, and the prevalence rate is approximately 1%. RA can occur at any age, increasing with age and peaking between the ages of 35 and 50 years [10]. RA affects all populations, though it is much more prevalent in some groups (e.g., 5%–6% in some Native American groups) and much less prevalent in others (e.g., black persons from the Caribbean region).

First-degree relatives of individuals with RA are at two- to three fold higher risk for the disease. Disease concordance in monozygotic twins is approximately 15%–20%, suggesting that nongenetic factors play an important role. Because the worldwide frequency of RA is relatively constant, a ubiquitous infectious agent has been postulated to play an etiologic role.

Women are affected by RA approximately 3 times more often than men are but sex differences diminish in older age groups. In investigating whether the higher rate of RA among women could be linked to certain reproductive risk factors, a study from Denmark found that the rate of RA was higher in women who had given birth to just one child than in women who had delivered two or three offspring [11]. However, the rate was not increased in women who were nulliparous or who had a history of lost pregnancies.

Time elapsed since pregnancy is also significant. In the one- to five-year postpartum period, a decreased risk for RA has been recognized, even in those with higher-risk HLA markers. The Danish study also found a higher risk of RA among women with a history of preeclampsia, hyperemesis during pregnancy, or gestational hypertension.

Etiology

1. **Genetic**: Exact cause is not known, although a genetic component appears likely. Genetic factors account for 50% of the risk for developing RA. About 60% of RA patients in the United States carry a shared epitope of the human leukocyte antigen (HLA)-DR4 cluster, which constitutes one of the peptide-binding sites of certain HLA-DR molecules associated with RA.
2. **Juvenile idiopathic arthritis (JIA)**, also known as juvenile rheumatoid arthritis (JRA), is a heterogeneous group of diseases that differs markedly from adult RA. JIA is known to have genetically complex traits in which multiple genes are important for disease onset and manifestations. It is characterized by arthritis

that begins before the age of 16 years, persists for more than 6 weeks, and is of unknown origin. The IL2RA/CD25 gene has been implicated as a JIA susceptibility locus, as has the VTCN1 gene.

3. **Infection**: For many decades, numerous infectious agents have been suggested as potential causes of RA, including Mycoplasma *o*rganisms, Epstein–Barr virus, and rubella virus. This suggestion is indirectly supported by the following evidence:
   - Occasional reports of flulike disorders preceding the start of arthritis
   - The inducibility of arthritis in experimental animals with different bacteria or bacterial products (e.g., streptococcal cell walls)
   - The presence of bacterial products, including bacterial RNA, in patients' joints
   - The disease-modifying activity of several agents that have antimicrobial effects, for example, gold salts, antimalarial agents, minocycline.
     Emerging evidence also points to an association between RA and periodontopathic bacteria. For example, the synovial fluid of RA patients has been found to contain high levels of antibodies to anaerobic bacteria that commonly cause periodontal infection, including *porphyromonasgingivalis.*

4. **Hormonal factors**: Women are more likely than men to develop RA, two to three times as many women as men. Sex hormones may play a role in RA, as evidenced by the disproportionate number of females with this disease, its amelioration during pregnancy, its recurrence in the early postpartum period, and its reduced incidence in women using oral contraceptives. Hyperprolactinemia may be a risk factor for RA.

5. **Immunologic factors**: All of the major immunologic elements play fundamental roles in initiating, propagating, and maintaining the autoimmune process of RA. The exact orchestration of the cellular and cytokine events that lead to pathologic consequences (e.g., synovial proliferation and subsequent joint destruction) is complex, involving T and B cells, antigen-presenting cells (APCs) (e.g., B cells, macrophages, and dendritic cells [DCs]), and various cytokines. Aberrant production and regulation of both proinflammatory and antiinflammatory cytokines and cytokine pathways are found in RA. The autoimmune response leads to the formation of immune complexes that activate the inflammatory process to a much higher degree than normal [12]. This theory is supported by the much worse prognosis of RA among patients with positive RF results.
   Factors that may increase your risk of RA include
   - **Smoking**: Cigarette smoking increases your risk of developing RA, particularly if you have a genetic predisposition for developing the disease. Smoking also appears to be associated with greater disease severity.
   - **Environmental exposures**: Although poorly understood, some exposures such as asbestos or silica may increase the risk of developing RA. Emergency workers exposed to dust from the collapse of the World Trade Center are at higher risk of autoimmune diseases such as RA.

- **Obesity**: People—especially women age 55 and younger—who are over-weight or obese appear to be at a somewhat higher risk of developing RA.
- **Trauma or injury**: such as bone breakage or fracture, dislocation of a joint, and ligament damage

Pathogenesis

There are two major subtypes of RA according to the presence or absence of antici-trullinated protein antibodies (ACPAs). Citrullination is catalyzed by the calcium-dependent enzyme peptidyl-arginine-deiminase (PAD), changing a positively charged arginine to a polar but neutral citrulline as the result of a posttranslational modification. ACPAs can be detected in approximately 67% of RA patients and serve as a useful diagnostic reference for patients with early, undifferentiated arthritis and provide an indication of likely disease progression through to RA. The ACPA-positive subset of RA has a more aggressive clinical phenotype compared to ACPA-negative subset of RA. It is reported that ACPA-negative RA has different genetic association patterns and differential responses of immune cells to citrullinated antigens from those of ACPA-positive subset.

Triggering stage

The appearance of ACPA is now widely used to diagnose and predict RA due to its high specificity (>97%) in clinical practice. ACPA occurs as a result of an abnormal antibody response to a range of citrullinated proteins, including fibrin, vimentin, fibronectin, Epstein—Barr Nuclear Antigen 1 (EBNA-1), α-enolase, type II collagen, and histones, all of which are distributed throughout the whole body. ACPA production has been associated with genetic and environmental factors. The strongest genetic risk factor associated with ACPA-positive RA is found in genes encoding HLA-DR, especially HLA-DR1 and HLA-DR4, also known as "shared epitopes" (SEs) [13].

The environment acts as a triggering factor for ACPA production in RA and the epigenetic regulation combines environment with genes. Gene—environment interaction influences the reactivity of autoantibodies to citrullinated antigens in RA. ACPAs can be detected long before the onset of the joint symptoms. This phenomenon suggests that the joints may not be the triggering spot for autoimmunity. Lung exposure to noxious agents, including smoke, silica dust, nanosized silica, or carbon-derived nanomaterials can trigger mucosal toll-like receptors that activate Ca^{2+} mediated PADs, but also APCs, such as classical DCs and B cells.

Maturation stage

This stage is initiated at the site of secondary lymphoid tissues or bone marrow. Epitope spreading refers to the development of immune responses to endogenous epitopes resulting from the release of self-antigens. The immune response to autoantigens may exist many years before disease onset and lay outside the joints. In this stage, epitope spreading and a gradually increased titer of ACPA can last several years before the onset of joint symptoms.

Targeting stage

The involvement of RA in joints usually has a characteristic presentation with synovitis occurring in symmetrical small joints. Joint swelling is the external reflection of synovial membrane inflammation following immune activation. Many cells and their cytokines play critical roles in the development of RA. The synovial compartment is infiltrated by leukocytes and the synovial fluid is inundated with proinflammatory mediators that are produced to induce an inflammatory cascade, which is characterized by interactions of fibroblast-like synoviocytes (FLSs) with the cells of the innate immune system, including monocytes, macrophages, mast cells, DCs, and so on, as well as cells of adaptive immune system such as T cells and B cells. Endothelial cells contribute to the extensive angiogenesis.

Fulminant stage

The fulminant stage contains hyperplastic synovium, cartilage damage, bone erosion, and systemic consequence. Bone resorption virtually creates bone erosions, which are usually found at spots where the synovial membrane inserts into the periosteum, which is known as a bare area according to certain anatomical features. The destruction of the subchondral bone can eventually result in the degeneration of the articular cartilage as the result of a decrease in osteoblasts and an increase in osteoclasts and synoviocytes.

Hyperplastic synovium: Synovium is characterized by a mixture of bone marrow-derived macrophages and specialized FLSs. Synovial cells maintain the steady state of the joint by secreting hyaluronic acid and lubricin for joint lubrication and function, as well as processing waste products. In RA, the dysfunction of FLS leads to hyperplastic synovium. The abnormal proliferation of FLS results from a loss of contact inhibition that plays a critical role in RA by producing inflammatory cytokines and proteinases, such as matrix metalloproteinases and tissue inhibitors of metalloproteinases that perpetuate joint destruction. They create a microenvironment that allows for the survival of T cell and B cell and neutrophil accumulation.

Cartilage damage: Cartilage acts as a key component of synovial joints, consisting of chondrocytes and a dense highly organized extracellular matrix synthesized by these chondrocytes and contains type II collagen and glycosaminoglycans. The hyperplastic synovium causes major damage to the cartilage in RA through directed adhesion and invasion.

Bone erosion: Bone loss is a pathological hallmark of RA and manifests as localized, periarticular, and systemic bone loss. Bone loss is the result of the induction of osteoclasts and the suppression of osteoblasts. "Periarticular" bone loss most likely refers to cellular changes of the subchondral bone marrow, such as osteoclast differentiation and the formation of inflammatory infiltrates.

Systemic consequences: Multiple studies have documented an elevated risk of cardiovascular events in RA patients. The mechanisms responsible for this risk may be related to cytokines that increase endothelial activation and potentially make atheromatous plaques unstable. Patients with active untreated RA have reduced total cholesterol, low-density, and high-density cholesterol. RA also influences the brain by causing fatigue and reduced cognitive function; the lungs by causing inflammatory and fibrotic disease; the exocrine glands by causing secondary Sjogren's syndrome; the skeletal muscles by causing sarcopenia; and the bones by causing osteoporosis. Rheumatoid nodules in 25%, usually those with severe disease in skin subject to pressure (ulnar forearm, elbows, occiput, lumbosacral area); also present in viscera; firm, nontender, with central fibrinoid necrosis surrounded by palisading epithelioidhistiocytes, lymphocytes, plasma cells; obliterative endarteritis in vasa nervorum and digital arteries causes ulcers, neuropathy, gangrene. Finally, RA patients may be at greater risk of cancer, especially hematologic and kidney cancers.

Signs and symptoms

Signs and symptoms of RA may include tender, warm, swollen joints, joint stiffness that is usually worse in the mornings and after inactivity, fatigue, fever, and loss of appetite.

Early RA tends to affect smaller joints of hands and feet. As the disease progresses, symptoms often spread to the wrists, knees, ankles, elbows, hips, and shoulders. In most cases, symptoms occur in the same joints on both sides of your body. About 40% of the people who have RA also experience signs and symptoms that don't involve the joints. RA can affect many structures other than the joints including skin, eyes, lungs, heart, kidneys, salivary glands, nerve tissue, bone marrow, blood vessels.

RA signs and symptoms may vary in severity and may even come and go. Periods of increased disease activity, called flares, alternate with periods of relative remission—when the swelling and pain fade or disappear.

Early signs

The main symptoms of RA are joint pain and stiffness. Before these symptoms occur, a person may experience some early warning signs.

1. **Fatigue**: Before experiencing any other symptoms, a person with RA may feel extremely tired and lack energy that may affect their everyday activities, relationships, sex drive, productivity at work, etc. They may also feel depressed.
2. **Slight fever**: Inflammation associated with RA may cause people to feel unwell and feverish.

3. **Weight loss**: An early warning sign of RA is unexplained weight loss probably due to loss of appetite.
4. **Stiffness**: Persistent stiffness, tenderness, and pain in joints may be an early sign of RA.
5. **Joint tenderness**: Joint tenderness that affects the hands and feet is a typical early sign of RA.
6. **Joint pain**: Joint pain in the fingers, wrists, and feet is a sign of RA. Inflammation makes the lining of the joint thicker and also causes the production of synovial fluid. It put pressure on the capsule that surrounds the joint and irritates the nerve endings that it contains, causing pain.
7. **Joint swelling**: Joints that look swollen in the hands and feet is a typical sign of RA. Joint swelling tends to be more apparent as RA progresses, but subtle swelling may be an early sign.
8. **Joint redness**: Inflammation in the joints may give them a red appearance. Discoloration of the skin around the joints in the hands and feet is a sign of RA. Redness occurs because the inflammation causes vasodilatation and increased circulation to the part.
9. **Joint warmth**: Joint warmth is caused by inflammation and may be present before redness or swelling occurs. This can be an early sign of RA.
10. **Numbness and tingling**: Numbness and tingling affecting the hands and feet may be an early sign of RA. These symptoms are caused by inflammation in the joints that can cause nerve compression, resulting in loss of sensation.
11. **Decrease in range of motion**: In the early stages of RA, a person may notice they are having trouble bending their wrist back and forth. As the disease progresses, damage to the joints can affect ligaments and tendons, making it hard to bend and straighten them.
12. **Joints affected on both sides**: It is common for people affected by RA to experience bilateral symmetrical symptoms.

Hand: The metacarpo-phalangeal (MCP) joints, proximal interphalangeal (PIP) joints, wrist joints including the carpometacarpal joint, midcarpal joint, radiocarpal joint, and intercarpal joints are often affected by RA. The distal interphalangeal (DIP) joints, of the fingers and thumb are affected by RA less frequently. When DIP joints are affected, it is typically only after symptoms appear in the MCP or PIP joints. It is more common for DIP joints to be affected by osteoarthritis than by RA.

Two common deformities of metacarpo-phalangeal joint associated with RA are palmer subluxation and ulnar drift. Z-deformity of thumb includes flexion of CMCJ with hyperextension of metacarpo-phalangeal joint and flexion of interphalangeal joint. Over time, damage to joints, tendons, and ligaments can cause bones to become malaligned, resulting in hand deformities.

Swan-neck deformity is characterized by flexion of DIP joint and hyperextension of PIP joint, is due to laxity or damage to volar plate. The collateral slips slip dorsally and hyperextends the PIP joint.

Treatment may include

- Finger splints or ring splints
- Surgery to realign the joints or fuse the joints so they work better

Boutonniere deformity, also called buttonhole deformity is characterized by flexion of PIP joint and hyperextension of DIP joint, is due to damage to central slip of extensor expansion. Flexion of PIP joint occurs by the unopposed action of FDS and the collateral slips slip volarly to hyperflex the PIP joint.

Tenosynovitis in the Hands: In addition to encapsulating joints, RA can affect tendon's synovial sheath, called tenosynovitis. The inflammation is not always painful but can lead to tendon damage. Tenosynovitis of flexor tendons in the hand may lead to **trigger finger** [14].

Wrist: About 75% of patients with RA develop wrist problems during the course of the disease. Synovitis begins in carpo-metacarpal joints followed by dorsal subluxation of metacarpal base. Destruction of carpals gives rise to radial deviation of wrist. Dislocation of inferior radio-ulnar joint with dorsal prominence of ulnar head and volar subluxation of ECU also occur.

Ankle & foot: About 20% of patients with RA the disease start from ankle and foot. Clawing of toes and hammer toe deformities, dislocation of metatarsophalangeal joints, hallux valgus and severe cases flat foot with broadening of forefoot develops. Achilles tendinitis, rheumatoid nodules are seen on ball of toes, side of foot and toes, bunion occurs when the great toe dislocates.

HIP joint: RA of the hip joint is less common, but it may occur as a later symptom in up to 28% of people with RA. It may affect one or both hips. It may be the only joint affected by RA. As with other joints, one will probably notice morning pain and stiffness. However, morning stiffness improves with movement or activity. Overtime develops dull aching pain that spreads to the groin, thigh, or buttock, pain that gets worse with walking or standing, pain even when resting. Patient walks with a limp. Hip pain doesn't always indicate RA. Hip pain may starts as mild and intermittent. One may only feel discomfort at the end of certain weight-bearing activities such as walking, jogging, hiking, weight training, dancing, climbing stairs, playing tennis, etc. But as the disease progresses and damages the hip joint, pain becomes more regular or constant. Discomfort may continue while at rest or sleeping. Pain in the hip joint can also make it difficult to stand or walk.

Knee: RA knee starts with synovitis and joint swelling. This causes pain from the inflammation of the tissue and knee movement is also limited. This makes it difficult or impossible to walk or stand without pain or weakness. Over time, the swelling can damage the cartilage and ligaments of the knee joints followed by subchondral bone damage. There occurs knee flexion with genu valgum or varum deformity. Windswept deformities are also seen.

Shoulder: RA affecting the shoulder region is a progressive disorder that results in pain, loss of range of motion, and functional disability. The inflammatory response results in synovitis, pannus formation, and articular destruction. Rotator cuff degeneration secondary to synovitis may limit abduction and rotation. Superolateral migration of the humerus occurs with complete tears.

Spine: Cervical spine is affected in the later stage and less frequently. Synovitis of atlanto-occipital and atlanto-axial joints and erosion occurs over time. Atlanto-axial subluxation occurs in 65%, superior odontoid migration occurs in 20% and 15% subaxial subluxation of all cervical involvement. Anterior subluxation occurs in 70% cases, lateral subluxation in 20%, posterior subluxation in about 07% and rotational subluxation is rare. Subluxation endangers the spinal cord with high cord compression and quadriparesis.

Extraarticular manifestations in RA are a serious condition, and RA patients with extraarticular manifestations should be aggressively treated and monitored.

Skin: Rheumatoid nodules are the most frequent skin manifestations (20%) in RA. They occur mainly in rheumatoid factor positive RA patients and in early RA give risk to severe extraarticular manifestations. Histologically focal central fibrinoid necrosis with surrounding fibroblasts is observed: it is believed to occur as a result of small vessel vasculitis. Other manifestations of rheumatoid small vessel vasculitis affecting the skin are splinter hemorrhages, periungual infarcts, leg ulcers, digital gangrene ,and sharply demarcated painful ulcerations. They appear mostly at the lower extremities or where skin is exposed to pressure.

Eyes: The most frequent is kerato-conjunctivitis-sicca, which affects at least 10% of patients. It is frequently observed together with xerostomia in a secondary Sjögren's syndrome.

Oral: Oral dryness and salivary gland swelling can also be found in patients with RA. These patients can also develop secondary Sjögren's syndrome.

GI system: Gastrointestinal complications in RA are mostly iatrogenic and caused by medications. Primary involvement of the gastrointestinal tract, caused by mesenteric vasculitis leading to intestinal infarction, is very rare. This condition causes acute abdominal pain, and can lead to intestinal bleeding and perforation.

Pulmonary: Pulmonary involvement in RA is frequent although not always clinically recognized. Pleural disease is common but usually asymptomatic; autopsy studies reported pleural involvement in 50% of cases, with only 10% clinically detected. Pleural effusions are usually exudates with mixed cell counts and high protein concentration. The disease is frequently associated with exudative pericarditis, and with interstitial lung disease. Parenchymal pulmonary nodules generally are asymptomatic and found in RF-positive patients with nodules elsewhere [15].

Cardiac: RA patients are also more prone to heart conditions like the thickening of the artery walls (atherosclerosis) and heart attacks. Extraarticular manifestations of RA and the presence of traditional cardiovascular risk factors were also found. The risk for myocardial infarction in female RA patients is twice that of women without RA, and in long-standing disease of at least 10 years, the risk is 3 times higher. Pericarditis is the most common cardiac manifestation in RA Congestive heart failure may be more frequent and is clinically evident in RA. Endocarditis with formation of rheumatoid nodules in the aortic or mitral valves can lead to valvular dysfunction.

Renal: Renal involvement in RA is rare, mesangial glomerulonephritis was the most common histopathological finding, whereas amyloidosis was the most common finding among patients with nephritic syndrome.

Neurological: Peripheral neuropathy, presenting as diffuse sensorimotor neuropathy or mononeuritis multiplex, occurs in a small subset of patients with RA. The underlying mechanism is small vessel vasculitis of the vasa vasorum of the nerves with ischemic neuropathy and demyelination. Cervical myelopathy, caused by atlantoaxial subluxation or pannus formation, occurs frequently in RA patients with severe and longstanding disease.

Hematological: Patients with RA may present with hematological abnormalities either at the time of diagnosis, or during the course of their illness. Hematological manifestations in RA can be broadly categorized into areas of anemia, neutropenia, thrombocytopenia, thrombocytosis, eosinophilia, and hematological malignancies.

Complications

RA increases your risk of developing:

- **Osteoporosis**: RA itself, along with some medications used for treating RA, can increase your risk of osteoporosis—a condition that weakens your bones and makes them more prone to fracture.
- **Rheumatoid nodules**: These firm bumps of tissue most commonly form around pressure points, such as the elbows. However, these nodules can form anywhere in the body, including the lungs.
- **Dry eyes and mouth**: People who have RA are much more likely to experience Sjogren's syndrome, a disorder that decreases the amount of moisture in your eyes and mouth.
- **Infections**: The disease itself and many of the medications used to combat RA can impair the immune system, leading to increased infections.
- **Abnormal body composition**: The proportion of fat to lean mass is often higher in people who have RA, even in people who have a normal body mass index.
- **Carpal tunnel syndrome**: If RA affects your wrist, the inflammation can compress the nerve that serves most of your hand and fingers.
- **Heart problems**: RA can increase your risk of hardened and blocked arteries, as well as inflammation of the sac that encloses your heart.
- **Lung disease**: People with RA have an increased risk of inflammation and scarring of the lung tissues, which can lead to progressive shortness of breath.
- **Lymphoma**: RA increases the risk of lymphoma, a group of blood cancers that develop in the lymph system.

Diagnosis

RA can be difficult to diagnose because it can mimic other diseases like lupus and fibromyalgia, in the early stage. Knowing your family history is also helpful because genetics may play a role in this disease. There isn't one single test to diagnose this condition. Even so, blood tests can check for autoantibodies and for markers of inflammation. These tests include

- **Rheumatoid factor test**: The RF blood test checks for a protein called rheumatoid factor. High levels of rheumatoid factor are associated with autoimmune diseases, especially RA.
- **Anticitrullinated protein antibody test (anti-CCP)**: This test looks for an antibody that's associated with RA. People who have this antibody usually have the disease. However, not everyone with RA tests positive for this antibody. The anti-CCP Ab is more specific for RA than the RF test
- **Antinuclear antibody test**: The antinuclear antibody panel tests your immune system to see if it's producing antibodies. Your body may make antibodies as a response to many different types of conditions, including RA.
- **Erythrocyte sedimentation rate**: The ESR test helps determine the degree of inflammation in your body. The result tells your doctor whether inflammation is present. However, it doesn't indicate the cause of the inflammation.
- **C-reactive protein test**: A severe infection or significant inflammation anywhere in your body can trigger your liver to make C-reactive protein. High levels of this inflammatory marker are associated with RA.
- **Imaging tests** are also used to detect inflammation and joint damage includes X-ray, MRI, or ultrasound, Bone scan.

Types of rheumatoid arthritis

Seropositive RA is characterized by a positive rheumatoid factor blood test result. This means you have the antibodies that cause your immune system to attack joints. Seropositive RA is the most common type of RA. This type of arthritis may run in families. Seropositive RA may come with more severe symptoms than seronegative RA. Presenting symptoms of seropositive RA can include morning stiffness lasting 30 min or longer, swelling and pain in multiple joints, bilaterally symmetrical joints involvement, rheumatoid nodules, fever, fatigue, weight loss, etc. Some people with seropositive RA can experience inflammation in the eyes, salivary glands, nerves, kidneys, lungs, heart, skin, and blood vessels.

Seronegative RA is characterized by a negative RF blood test result and a negative anti-CCP result, but one still has RA symptoms. One may eventually develop antibodies, changing your diagnosis to seropositive RA.

JIA refers to RA in children ages 17 years old and younger. The condition was previously known as JRA. The symptoms are the same as those of other types of RA, but they may also include eye inflammation and issues with physical development.

Treatment

There's no cure for RA, but there are treatments that can help you manage it. RA can keep both patients and physicians on their toes as they figure out the best ways to treat the symptoms and slow the progression of the condition. Recently, advances in treatment strategies have resulted in ever-improving outcomes and quality of life for those with RA. Treat to Target RA is a treatment philosophy that rheumatologists use to effectively manage this disease.The treat-to-target approach has resulted in fewer symptoms and higher remission rates for those with RA. The treatment strategy involves setting a specific testing goal that signals either remission or low disease state, testing acute phase reactants, and performing monthly monitoring to assess progress of treatment and management plan, switching medication regimen promptly if progress isn't made [16].

Treatments for RA help to manage the pain and control the inflammatory response which can in many cases result in remission. Decreasing the inflammation can also help to prevent further joint and organ damage.

Treatments—It may include medications, physiotherapy, dietary changes, and life style modifications. For many people, these treatments help them live an active life and reduce the risk of long-term complications.

Medications:There are many types of medication for RA. Some of these medications help to reduce the pain and inflammation of RA. Some help to reduce flares and limit the damage that RA does to your joints.Non-steroidal anti-inflammatory drugs (NSAIDs), corticosteroids, acetaminophen, Disease-modifying antirheumatic drugs (DMARDs) help reduce the pain and inflammation during RA flares.

A number of medications can be used to treat RA. Those include

- **OTC pain relievers**: If symptoms are mild, over-the-counter nonsteroidal antiinflammatory medications can help manage inflammation and pain. These include ibuprofen (Motrin) and naproxen sodium (Aleve).
- **Corticosteroids**: These are very effective at reducing pain and inflammation. Steroids are available orally, or your doctor can administer a steroid injection in your hip. Your doctor may prescribe a corticosteroid for a brief period for severe flares, or as a bridge until other medication is effective. They're not recommended as a long-term treatment due to side effects.
- **DMARDs**: DMARDs decrease inflammation and stop the progression of RA. Options include methotrexate (Trexall), leflunomide (Arava), tofacitinib (Xeljanz), or hydroxychloroquine (Plaquenil).
- **Biologics**: If the above therapies aren't effective, your doctor may recommend a biologic or targeted therapy. This newer class of antirheumatic drugs works by targeting specific parts of the immune system that trigger an inflammatory response. Biologics can be used alone or combined with other DMARDs.
- **Janus kinase (JAK) inhibitors**: These are a new subcategory of DMARDs that block certain immune responses. These are drugs that your healthcare provider may use to help prevent inflammation and stop damage to your joints when DMARDs and biologic DMARDs don't work for you.

Diet: Dietician may recommend an antiinflammatory diet to help with your symptoms. This type of diet includes foods that have lots of omega-3 fatty acids. Foods high in omega-3 fatty acids include fatty fish like salmon, tuna, herring, and mackerel, chia seeds, flax seeds, walnuts, etc. Antioxidants, such as vitamins A, C, and E, and selenium, may also help reduce inflammation. Foods high in antioxidants include berries, such as blueberries, cranberries, goji berries, and strawberries, dark chocolate, spinach, kidney beans, pecans, artichokes, etc. Eating lots of fiber is also important. According to some researchers, fiber may help reduce inflammatory responses which may decrease C-reactive protein levels. Choose whole grain foods, fresh vegetables, and fresh fruit. Strawberries may be particularly beneficial. Foods containing flavonoids can also help to counter inflammation in the body. They include soy products, such as tofu and miso, berries, green tea, broccoli, grapes, etc. What you don't eat is just as important as what you do eat. Make sure to avoid trigger foods. These include processed carbohydrates and saturated or trans-fats. Avoiding trigger foods and choosing the right foods in trying to follow an anti-inflammatory diet may help you manage your RA.

Prognosis

Outcome in RA is compromised when diagnosis and treatment are delayed. The clinical course of RA is generally one of exacerbations and remissions. Approximately 40% of patients with this disease become disabled after 10 years, but outcomes are highly variable. Some patients experience a relatively selflimited disease, whereas others have a chronic progressive illness.

Prognostic factors: Intervention with DMARDs in very early RA (symptom duration <12 weeks at the time of first treatment) provides the best opportunity for achieving disease remission. Better detection of early joint injury has provided a previously unappreciated view of the ubiquity and importance of early joint damage. Nonetheless, predicting the long-term course of an individual case of RA at the outset remains difficult, though the following all correlate with an unfavorable prognosis in terms of joint damage and disability—HLA-DRB1*04/04 genotype, high serum titer of auto-antibodies (e.g., RF and ACPA), extraarticular manifestations, large number of involved joints, age younger than 30 years, female sex, systemic symptoms, and insidious onset.

The prognosis of RA is generally much worse among patients with positive RF results. For example, the presence of RF in sera has been associated with severe erosive disease. However, the absence of RF does not necessarily portend a good prognosis.

RA that remains persistently active for longer than 1 year is likely to lead to joint deformities and disability. Periods of activity lasting only weeks or a few months followed by spontaneous remission portend a better prognosis.

A study by Mollard et al. of 8189 women in a US-wide observational cohort who developed RA before menopause found greater functional decline in postmenopausal women than in premenopausal ones; furthermore, the trajectory of functional decline worsened and accelerated after menopause [17]. However, ever-use of hormonal replacement therapy, ever having a pregnancy, and longer length of reproductive life were associated with less functional decline.

Physiotherapy

Physical therapy can help you learn ways to move without pain or injury. Occupational therapy is helpful to learn easier ways to perform activities of daily living, such as dressing, cooking, eating, or cleaning.

Exercises

- Rest is best during flare-upstage. Getting enough sleep will help to reduce inflammation and pain as well as fatigue. Regular exercise is important for RA. Low-impact exercises can help to improve the range of motion in the joints and increase mobility. Exercise can also strengthen muscles, which can help to relieve some of the pressure from the joints. Strengthening, endurance, flexibility, and mobility exercises are important to prevent painful falls, deep breathing exercises and relaxation. These can all help lessen stress. Chronic stress stimulates your body to produce more mediators of inflammation throughout your body.
- **Low-impact exercises.** This may help to reduce inflammation and ease hip pain. Try gentle workouts, including walking, swimming, or water aerobics.
- Ice packs or cold compresses can help to reduce inflammation and pain. They may also be effective against muscle spasms. Contrast bath by alternate cold with hot treatments such as warm showers and hot compresses may help to reduce stiffness. Use heat to reduce stiffness in the joints.
- The aim of Physical therapy in treating hip RA is to maintain and increase range of motion and muscle strength. A cane, walker, or other assistive device may be provided to relieve stress and prevent or minimize further damage [18].
- If pain and disability continue to worsen despite treatment, total hip replacement may be the option. Total hip replacement relieves pain and restores motion. About 80% of the time is to maintain and increase range of motion and muscle strength

Try assistive devices: Certain devices such as splints and braces in a resting position can be given to rest the part that may help to reduce inflammation. Canes and crutches can help to relieve load on lower extremity joints while maintaining mobility, even during flares. Install household devices such as grab bars and handrails in bathrooms and along staircases is useful.

Home remedies for rheumatoid arthritis: Certain home remedies and lifestyle adjustments may help to improve your quality of life when living with RA. This includes exercise, rest, and assistive devices.

If RA in the hip limits mobility, working with a physical therapist or an occupational therapist can help improve joint flexibility and walking. You'll learn specific exercises to strengthen your hip joint. A few strategies include

Morbidity and mortality

Estimates suggest that more than 50% of these patients remain fully employed, even after 10−15 years of disease, with one-third having only intermittent low-grade disease and another one-third experiencing spontaneous remission.

RA is associated with traditional and nontraditional cardiovascular risk factors. The leading cause of excess mortality in RA is cardiovascular disease, followed by infection, respiratory disease, and malignancies. The effects of concurrent therapy, which is often immunosuppressive, may contribute to mortality in RA. However, studies suggest that control of inflammation may improve mortality.

Nontraditional risk factors appear to play an important role in cardiovascular morbidity and mortality. Myocardial infarction, myocardial dysfunction, and asymptomatic pericardial effusions are common; symptomatic pericarditis and constrictive pericarditis are rare. Myocarditis, coronary vasculitis, valvular disease, and conduction defects are occasionally observed. A large Danish cohort study suggested the presence of an increased risk of atrial fibrillation and stroke in patients with RA.

The overall mortality in patients with RA is reportedly 2.5 times higher than that of the general age-matched population. In the 1980s, mortality among those with severe articular and extraarticular disease approached that among patients with 3-vessel coronary disease or stage IV Hodgkin lymphoma. Much of the excess mortality derives from infection, vasculitis, and poor nutrition. With the exception of lymphoma, mortality from cancer is unchanged.

Patient Education: Patient education and counseling help to reduce pain, disability, and frequency of physician visits. These may represent the most cost-effective intervention for RA.

Informing patient of diagnosis

With a potentially disabling disease such as RA, the act of informing the patient of the diagnosis takes on major importance. The goal is to satisfy the patient's informational needs regarding the diagnosis, prognosis, and treatment in appropriate detail. To understand the patient's perspective, requests, and fears, the physician must employ careful questioning and empathetic listening.

Telling patients more than they are intellectually or psychologically prepared to handle (a common practice) risks making the experience so intense as to trigger withdrawal. Conversely, failing to address issues of importance to the patient compromises the development of trust. The patient needs to know that the primary physician understands the situation and is available for support, advice, and therapy as the need arises. Encouraging the patient to ask questions helps to communicate interest and caring.

Discussing prognosis and treatment

Patients and families do best when they know what to expect and can view the illness realistically. Many patients fear crippling consequences and dependency. Accordingly, it is valuable to provide a clear description of the most common disease manifestations. Without encouraging false hopes, the physician can point out that spontaneous remissions can occur and that more than two thirds of patients live independently without major disability [19]. In addition, emphasize that much can be done to minimize discomfort and to preserve function.

A review of available therapies and their efficacy helps patients to overcome feelings of depression stemming from an erroneous expectation of inevitable disability. Even in those with severe disease, guarded optimism is now appropriate, given the host of effective and well-tolerated disease-modifying treatments that are emerging.

Dealing with misconceptions

Several common misconceptions regarding RA deserve attention. Explaining that no known controllable precipitants exist helps to eliminate much unnecessary guilt and self-recrimination. Dealing in an informative, evidence-based fashion with a patient who expresses interest in alternative and complementary forms of therapy can help limit expenditures on ineffective treatments.

Another misconception is that a medication must be expensive to be helpful. Generic NSAIDs, low-dose prednisone and the first-line DMARDs are quite inexpensive yet remarkably effective for relieving symptoms, a point that bears emphasizing. The belief that one must be given the latest TNF inhibitor to be treated effectively can be addressed by a careful review of the overall treatment program and the proper role of such agents in the patient's plan of care.

Active participation of the patient and family in the design and implementation of the therapeutic program helps boost morale and to ensure compliance, as does explaining the rationale for the therapies used.

The family also plays an important part in striking the proper balance between dependence and independence. Household members should avoid overprotecting the patient (e.g., the spouse refraining from intercourse out of fear of hurting the patient) and should work to sustain the patient's pride and ability to contribute to the family. Allowing the patient with RA to struggle with a task is sometimes constructive.

Supporting patient with debilitating disease

Abandonment is a major fear in these individuals. Patients are relieved to know that they will be closely observed by the primary physician and healthcare team, working in conjunction with a consulting rheumatologist and physical/occupational therapist, all of whom are committed to maximizing the patient's comfort and independence and to preserving joint function. With occupational therapy, the treatment effort is geared toward helping the patient maintain a meaningful work role within the limitations of the illness.

Persons with long-standing severe disease who have already sustained much irreversible joint destruction benefit from an emphasis on comfort measures, supportive counseling, and attention to minimize further debility. Such patients need help in grieving for their disfigurement and loss of function.

Traumatic conditions

Fracture neck of femur

Fracture neck of femur is intracapsular and is the commonest fracture in elderly persons. Neck of femur is relatively weaker due to poor trabecular system. In elderly persons, it becomes weaker due to senile osteoporosis, more so in elderly female due to menopausal osteoporosis [1]. Fracture neck of femur occurs due to fall, relatively more common due to fall in the bathroom from slippage of the foot. Simple stumbling may also result in fracture neck of femur. Fracture neck of femur in younger people occurs due to high energy trauma such as vehicle collision or fall from a great height. Fracture neck of femur is rare in children.

About 90% of the fracture neck of femur the distal fracture fragment is displaced upward by the pull of glutei attached to greater trochanter and rotated externally by the pull of strong hip external rotators attached to medial aspect of the greater trochanter. There is shortening and external rotation attitude [2]. One finds inability to bear the load. In about 10% of cases, the fracture is impacted and becomes stable. One can get up unaided and bear load with some discomfort. There are no shortening and hip movements are possible with some discomfort.

Since fracture neck of femur is intracapsular, the hemorrhagic fluid flushed with synovial fluid and doesn't clot. The absence of hematoma formation, which is the first stage of fracture healing leads to fracture nonunion. The fracture site doesn't directly come in contact with the soft tissue, which is another factor for fracture nonunion. If at all the fracture heals it may heal with malunion, that is, supratrochanteric shortening with limb length discrepancy and external rotation of the limb.

The head of the femur is supplied by nutrient artery, circumflex femoral arteries, and artery accompanying ligamentum teres. In case of fracture neck of femur, the nutrient artery and circumflex femoral arteries which are the main source of blood supply to head of femur may get damaged as they are intimately related to neck of the femur. Higher is the fracture site more is the chance of injury to the arteries. The only artery remain is artery accompanying ligamentum teres, which is insufficient to keep the head of the femur alive. So, it leads to avascular necrosis of head of femur.

Fracture neck of femur can be classified into subcapital, cervical, and basal. Higher is the fracture site more is the chance of nonunion and avascular necrosis of head of femur.

Elderly persons with history of fall, pain in the groin and thigh, finds difficulty to get up and bear weight, the limb is externally rotated with shortening, no active movement is possible is diagnostic of fracture neck of femur. X-rays confirms the diagnosis.

Garden classification is based on X-rays AP view. Type I—incomplete, that is, valgus impacted, Type II—complete but undisplaced, Type III—complete and partially displaced, Type IV—complete and fully displaced.

Management

As a rule, fracture neck of femur is managed by open reduction internal fixation by Smith Peterson's nailing/dynamic compression screw plate/two to three cannulated screw/sliding hip screw. In nondisplaced fracture, percutaneous cannulated screws or sliding hip screw is used. However, there is higher risk of avascular necrosis with sliding hip screw than cannulated screws. Replacement arthroplasty is indicated in elderly patients. Hemiarthroplasty is indicated in less active patients, whereas total hip arthroplasty is indicated in more active patients.

Postoperative PT

It is always active. The aim is to restore preaccidental, even better than that condition. The part is given rest in neutral rotation and slight abduction. Adduction and rotation movement are contraindicated as it may loosen the fixation. Immediate postoperatively active ankle, foot, toe movements should be given to prevent deep vein thrombosis. Chest PT includes deep breathing exercise, effective huffing and coughing to prevent chest complications.

Active assisted hip, knee flexion-extension by sliding the heel on the couch can start from second day. Active assisted abduction from abducted position starts from 3 to 4 day. Progressive ROM exercise should be given so that by seventh day full ROM should be achieved. Static quadriceps, static gluteal, ankle-foot-toe movements should be practiced regularly. The intrinsic muscles exercises include toe parting and closing, foot shortening, and elongation against a foot support to prevent flat foot.

Static gluteal exercise, quadriceps start from third day, assisted hip knee flexion-extension, abduction starts from second day. So that by 5–7 days active free hip knee flexion-extension should be possible. No resistance should be given. One can practice nonweight bearing walking by the walker once postoperative pain subsides. Progressive resisted exercise and partial weight bearing walking starts after 6 weeks.

Straight leg raising can be initiated with assistance from second to third day provided the hip is not stiff; otherwise, movements occur at the fracture site rather than the stiff hip joint. Turning every 2 hourly through the sound side should be encouraged while holding the operated limb in slight abduction.

Patient is made to sit in the bed from second to third day. Standing in nonweight bearing starts from fifth day. Patient is discharged once he learns nonweight bearing walking. He reports after 6 weeks, so that progressive resisted exercise and partial weight bearing walking can be initiated. Again, patient reports after 3 weeks to start full weight bearing.

Complications

1. **Fracture nonunion**: About one-fourth to one-third of the cases with fracture neck of femur develop nonunion [3]. Overtime the neck gets absorbed and the head sinks toward the trochanter. Loosening of the internal fixator occurs resulting in redisplacement of fracture fragment. Patient complains of acute pain. There occur shortening and external rotation of limb and one finds inability to walk.

2. **Avascular necrosis of head of femur (AVN)**: Avascular necrosis (or Osteonecrosis) is a condition affecting the femoral head. Damage to the nutrient artery and circumflex femoral arteries compromises circulation to head of femur predisposing to avascular necrosis of head of femur. Once the bone dies, the femoral head collapses and if severe enough, the hip joint itself collapses. One complains of acute pain, weakness around the hip and unable to bear the load. **Management of AVN**—Provide walking aids to protect head from further damage. Mobilization of stiff hip and progressive strengthening of muscles around hip should be given carefully.

3. **Osteoarthritis of hip**: Damage to the articular surface of head of femur due to AVN predisposes to secondary OA of hip. It can be managed by gentle joint mobilization and progressive strengthening of muscle around joint.

4. **Fracture Mal-union**: Fracture neck of femur unites with external rotation and shortening.

Nonoperative management is indicated in nonambulatory patients, minimal pain, and those who are at high risk for surgery. Derotational boot and skin traction is given.

Fracture trochanter

Incidence of fracture greater trochanter is more than that of fracture neck of femur. Fracture neck of femur is intracapsular, whereas fracture trochanter is extracapsular (Fig. 5.1). Fracture is more common in elderly person and caused due to fall. It may be subtrochanteric or intertrochanteric [4].

Subtrochanteric fracture: A subtrochanteric region is defined as within 5 cm distal to the lesser trochanter. Subtrochanteric fracture in elderly with osteoporosis occurs due to trivial injury, whereas in young population occurs in high energy mechanisms such as motor vehicle collisions. The proximal fragment with head

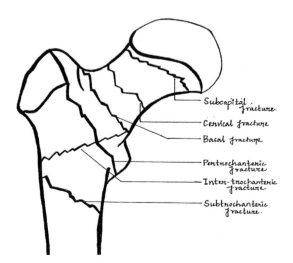

FIGURE 5.1

Classification of fracture neck of femur and fracture trochanter.

and neck of femur is abducted, externally rotated by the strong pull of glutei and external rotators, flexed by the iliopsoas. It may threaten skin anteriorly. The distal fragment is held shortened and in adduction due to pull of adductors on medial femoral condyle [5].

According to Russel-Taylor classification, Type-I: fracture extends into piriformis fossa that is amenable to an intramedullary nail and Type-II: fracture extends into greater trochanter with involvement of piriformis fossa as seen on X-rays lateral view that is treated by fixed angle plate [6].

Blood loss is more in subtrochanteric fracture than fracture neck of femur and intertrochanteric fracture. Complains of pain hip and thigh that aggravate with hip movement. There is marked swelling of thigh is present. There is shortening with external rotation of leg. One finds difficulty to get up and bear the load. Since fracture is extracapsular and the fracture site is highly vascular, it always unites readily. It heals with mal-union due to displacement following fracture.

Nonoperative treatment is indicated in nonambulatory patients with medical comorbidities that would not allow them to undergo surgery. Displacement due to strong muscle pull and deformities makes it difficult to make the patient walk without surgical fixation. Russel-Taylor type-I fracture is treated with intramedullary nail and type II fracture is treated with fixed 95° angle blade plate. Interlocking fixation is preferred. Blade plate may function as a tension band construct.

Complication of subtrochanteric fracture includes mal-union and coxavara.

Intertrochanteric fracture: Intertrochanteric fracture occurs between greater and lesser trochanter and composed of dense trabecular bone. Gluteus medius and minimus, hip external rotators such as obturators, gemelii, piriformis are attached to greater trochanter and iliopsoas is attached to lesser trochanter. Following fracture, the greater trochanter tends to displace upward and rotated externally, whereas the distal fracture fragment tends to flex. Intertrochanteric fracture in elderly persons with osteoporosis occurs due to low impact injury such as ground level fall and in younger population occurs from high impact injury such as road traffic accident or fall from greater height.

Fracture may be stable or unstable. Stable fractures have an intact posteromedial cortex. Unstable fractures include commoniton of posteromedial cortex, a thin lateral wall, and displaced lesser trochanter fracture. Evans classification of intertrochanteric fractures is based on displacement, number of fragments and type of fragment displaced. Type I is two segments fracture, Type II is three segments fracture, Type III is four segments fracture. It is further subclassified into A and B [7]. Type IA refers to nondisplaced and B displaced. In type IIA describes three segments fracture with separate greater trochanter fragment and B describes three segments fracture with a lesser trochanter fragment. In general, intertrochanteric fracture can be classified into stable and unstable fractures. Stable fractures are those in which the femur is broken into two or three parts. Unstable fractures are those in which the femur is broken into four parts including femoral head, lesser trochanter, greater trochanter, and remaining femur. Fracture line parallel to femoral neck is known as reverse oblique pattern, which is extremely unstable.

Complains of pain hip and thigh aggravate with hip movement. There is shortening with external rotation of leg. One finds difficulty to get up and bear the load. Since fracture is extracapsular and the fracture site is highly vascular, it always unites readily. It heals with mal-union due to displacement following fracture.

Nonoperative treatment is indicated in nonambulatory patients with medical comorbidities that would not allow them to undergo surgery. Sliding hip compression screw coupled to a side plate that is screwed into shaft of femur fixation is indicated in stable intertrochanteric fracture. Intramedullary nail is introduced through greater trochanter with distal locking and sliding hip screw is indicated in unstable intertrochanteric fracture. Comminution may make fixation with a sliding hip screw and side plate more likely to fail.

Complication of intertrochanteric fracture includes varus and rotational malunion. Supratrochanteric shortening with coxavara and external rotation, high riding GT limits hip abduction range due to premature bone contact, limping may be present due to inefficiency of hip abductor mechanism and shortening. Rarely nonunion occurs due to soft tissue interposition.

Postoperatively patient can be given rest in neutral rotation and slight abduction, immediately encourage deep breathing exercise, effective huffing and coughing, active ankle-foot-toe movement, turning at regular interval, etc. patient can be made to stand as early as possible with the help of walker. In case of rigid fixation standing on second or third day can be done and gradually nonweight bearing walking should be encouraged. Partial weight bearing starts after 8–10 weeks, full weight bearing after 12–14 weeks.

Fracture pelvis

Because the pelvis is a ring-like structure, a fracture in one part of the structure is often accompanied by a fracture or damage to ligaments at another point in the structure. Doctors have identified several common pelvic fracture patterns. The specific pattern of the fracture depends upon the direction in which it was broken and the amount of force that caused the injury.

Causes

1. **Trauma**: Pelvic fractures occur after both low-energy and high-energy events. The appearance of pelvic fractures is the greatest in people aged between 15 and 28 [8]. In persons, younger than 35, pelvic fractures occur more in males than in females. In persons, older than 35, pelvic fractures are more likely to happen to females than males. In younger people, pelvic fractures occur mostly as a result of high-energy mechanisms such as motor vehicle or motorcycle collision, crush accident, and falls from a significant height. Those high-energy pelvic fractures are one of the major injuries that lead to death. The presence of coma, shock, and head and chest injuries are predictors of death. In older people, they occur from minimal trauma, such as a low fall. Elderly people with osteoporosis have a higher risk factor. Low-energy fractures are usually stable fractures of the pelvic ring. Depending on the direction and magnitude of the force, these injuries can be life-threatening and require surgical treatment.
2. **Bone insufficiency**: A pelvic fracture may also occur due to osteoporosis in older people. In these patients, a fracture may occur even during a fall from standing or a routine activity such as getting out of the bathtub or descending stairs. These injuries are typically stable fractures that do not damage the structural integrity of the pelvic ring, but may fracture an individual bone.
3. **Other causes**: Less commonly, an avulsion fracture of the ischium bone may occur by the pull of hamstring muscles that is most common in young athletes who are still growing. An avulsion fracture does not usually make the pelvis unstable or injure internal organs.

In addition to being described by the specific fracture pattern, pelvic fractures are often described as "stable" or "unstable," based on how much damage has occurred to the structural integrity of the pelvic ring. Stable fracture: In this type of fracture, there is often only one break in the pelvic ring and the broken ends of the bones line up adequately. Low-energy fractures are often stable fractures. Stable pelvic fracture patterns include: Iliac wing fracture, sacrum fracture, superior and inferior pubic ramus fracture. Unstable fracture: In this type of fracture, there are usually two or more breaks in the pelvic ring and the ends of the broken bones do not line up correctly (displacement). This type of fracture is more likely to occur due to a high-energy event. Unstable pelvic fracture patterns include anterior-posterior compression fracture, lateral compression fracture -in this fracture, the pelvis is pushed inward, vertical shear fracture -in this fracture, one half of the pelvis shifts upward. Both stable and unstable pelvic fractures can also be divided into "open" fractures, in which the bone fragments stick out through the skin, or "closed" fractures, in which the skin is not broken. Open fractures are particularly serious because, once the skin is broken, infection in both the wound and the bone can occur. Immediate treatment is required to prevent infection.

Clinical features

A fractured pelvis is almost always painful that aggravates by moving the hip or attempting to walk. Often, the patient will try to keep his or her hip or knee bent in a specific position to avoid aggravating the pain. Some patients may experience swelling or bruising in the hip area. Pelvic fractures may be recognized by tenderness, pain, bruising, swelling, and crepitus of the pubis, iliac bones, hips, and sacrum. Physical findings could include abnormal position of the lower limbs and pelvic deformity or pelvic instability. With avulsion injuries, there is often pain associated with contraction of the involved muscles (Fig. 5.2).

There must be a differentiation between high impact unstable fractures and low impact stable pelvic fractures. This can be done by determination of the circumstances of the trauma. Patients with unstable fractures are usually unable to stand, in contrast to patients with stable fractures who can often walk unaided.

Pelvic fractures can be classified by several classification systems. Classification of pelvic fractures by Tile, which is most commonly used, is based on the integrity of the posterior sacroiliac complex [9].

1. Type A: rotationally and vertically stable, the sacroiliac complex is intact. Type A fractures are mostly managed nonoperatively.
   * A1:avulsion fractures.
   * A2: stable iliac wing fractures or minimally displaced pelvic ring fractures.
   * A3: transverse sacral or coccyx fractures.
2. Type B: rotationally unstable and vertically stable, caused by external or internal rotational forces, results in partial disruption of the posterior sacroiliac complex.

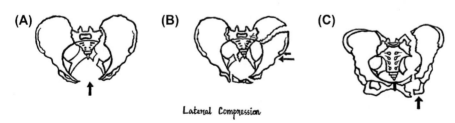

(A)

Antenoposterion Compression

(B)

Lateral Compression

(C)

Vertical Shear

FIGURE 5.2

Unstable pelvic fracture patterns a) antero-posterior compression b) lateral compression c) vertical shear.

- B1:open-book injuries.
- B2: lateral compression injuries.
- B3: bilateral rotational instability.

3. Type C: rotationally unstable and vertically unstable, complete disruption of the posterior sacroiliac complex. These unstable fractures are mostly caused by high-energy trauma like falls from height, motor vehicle accidents, or crushing injuries.
   - C1: unilateral injury.
   - C2: bilateral injuries in which one side is rotationally unstable and the contralateral side is vertically unstable.
   - C3: bilateral injury in which both sides are vertically unstable.

Seventy to 80 percent of all pelvic injuries are type A or type B fractures.

Emergency stabilization

Patients with high-energy fractures will almost always go or be brought to an urgent care center or emergency room for initial treatment due to the severity of their symptoms.

Other presenting factors are hematuria, rectal bleeding, hematoma, and neurological and vascular abnormalities in the legs. These patients may also have additional injuries to the head, chest, abdomen, or legs. If their injuries cause significant blood loss, it could lead to shock—a life-threatening condition that can result in organ failure.

The care of patients with high-energy pelvic fractures requires a multidisciplinary approach with input from a number of medical specialists. In some cases, airway, breathing, and circulatory problems must be addressed before treating the fracture and other injuries.

Physical examination

Because a high-energy trauma could damage the primary organ systems, the examination of a pelvic fracture should start with investigation of life-threatening injuries. The abdomen, perineum, genitals, rectum, and lower back must be examined very carefully. High-energy fractures are often associated with severe injuries of other organs. When life-threatening injuries are excluded, the examination should include an inspection and palpation of the pelvis to identify crepitus and to determine pelvic stability. It is necessary to examine whether related injuries are present. Some injuries that could be associated with pelvic injuries are: soft-tissue injuries, urethral injuries, skeletal injuries, neurovascular injuries and neurologic injuries.

Soft-tissue injuries like hematomas, abrasions, and lacerations commonly accompany pelvic ring injuries. Hematomas located at the scrotum, labium, flank, and the inguinal region are indicative of intrapelvic hemorrhage. Lacerations of the perineum, rectum, and vagina are indicative of severe injuries and could be indicative for contamination by urine or stool. Ohmori et al. concluded that the risk factors for massive hemorrhage are lactate level, AO/OTA classification, and pelvic extravasation of contrast fluid on CT. They created a new effective predictive score of massive hemorrhage in pelvic ring fractures. Pelvic fracture urethral injury is an uncommon but potentially devastating result of pelvic fracture. Symptoms of urethral injuries are blood at the external urethral meatus, a high-riding (nonpalpable) prostate gland in man, and perineal and genital swelling. Pelvic fractures often are present with bladder disruptions. The disruption may be intraperitoneal, extraperitoneal, or both. In patients with a bladder disruption gross, hematuria will be present.

Frequently pelvic fractures are associated with skeletal injuries. It is necessary that the clinician examines the spine and extremities. There could be limb length discrepancies, or internal/external rotational deformities.

Because many structures traverse the pelvis, it is possible that a pelvic injury causes injury to a neurovascular structure. Vascular injuries occur more often than arterial injuries. Both may contribute to hemorrhage. A vascular injury is very urgent to treat.

Sometimes there will also be neurological injuries. The nerve roots that are typically injured are L5 and S1. Sometimes L4 (severe pelvic injury) or S2–S5 nerves (sacral injuries) can be damaged too. The clinician should carefully detect these nerve injuries by a neurological examination.

Imaging studies—The diagnosis of a pelvic fracture mostly will be made by medical imaging. Imaging tests can determine the location of a fracture, how many bones are affected and whether an injury has damaged surrounding soft tissues, such as tendons, ligaments, blood vessels, or nerves:

- X-rays: antero-posterior view, inlet view, and outlet view.
- Computed tomography (CT) scans. Because of the complexity of this type of injury, a CT scan is commonly ordered for pelvic fractures. A CT scan will provide a more detailed, cross-sectional image of the pelvis and to better determine the specific pattern and extent of your injury, look for associated injuries, and aid in preoperative planning.
- Ultrasound
- Bone scans

The severity and correlated injuries can be investigated by Urinalysis, Measurement of hemoglobin and hematocrit to measure blood loss, retrograde urethrography, arteriography, cystography.

Treatment

Pelvic fractures should be considered in the context of a polytrauma management, rather than in isolation. The treatment and management of each patient requires careful, individualized decision making. Medical management of pelvic fractures consists, if necessary, resuscitation must be done then the patient and the fracture should be stabilized [10]. After the medical management is finished the rehabilitation can start.

The stabilization of pelvic fractures has historically been treated nonoperatively. Lately operative management has increased in the treatment of unstable pelvic fractures. Operative management of an unstable pelvic ring injury allows earlier mobilization, and thereby diminishes the complications of immobilization. Stabilization may also be important for the survival of the patient and may be desirable to improve the long-term functional results. It allows correction and prevention of significant pelvic deformities, so the clinical outcomes of the patient will improve.

In emergency, the fracture will be stabilized by an external fixator (for anteroposterior injuries) or a "C-clamp" (for vertical shear injuries). The definitive fixation can be done anteriorly or posteriorly and internal or external. Mostly plates or screws are used to stabilize a fracture. Rommens et al. concluded that more studies are needed to find the optimal treatment for each type of instability [11].

External fixation acts as a stabilizing frame to hold the broken bones in proper position. In some cases, an external fixator is used to stabilize the bones until healing is complete. In some cases, external fixator may be used as a temporary treatment until another procedure can be performed.

Other methods used to treat pelvic fractures are traction, spica casts, pelvic slings, and turnbuckles. Skeletal traction through femur or tibia is often used immediately after an injury and removed after surgery. Occasionally, acetabular fractures can be treated with skeletal traction alone.

Open reduction and internal fixation. During this operation, the displaced bone fragments are first reduced into their normal alignment and held together with screws or metal plates attached to the outer surface of the bone.

Physical therapy management

Physical therapy is an important part of the rehabilitation in both, low-energy and high-energy pelvic fractures. Low-energy injuries are usually managed with conservative care. This includes bed rest, pain control and physical therapy. High-energy injuries, especially the unstable fractures must be reduced by surgical treatment. Afterward physical therapy includes the same treatment as in low-energy fractures. Early mobilization is very important because prolonged immobilization can lead to many complications, including respiratory and circulatory dysfunctions. Physical therapy helps the patient to get out of bed as soon as possible.

Short-term goals for patients after surgery are independence with transfers and wheelchair mobility. Depending on the medical status of the patient these goals can be achieved in 2–6 weeks. The physical therapy program can be continued in the hospital or at home. The home-based program includes basic range of motion, stabilizing and strengthening exercises intended to prevent contracture and reduce atrophy.

The goals of the physical therapy program should provide the patient with an optimal return of function by improving functional skills, selfcare skills, and safety awareness. The main goals are to improve the pain level, strength, flexibility, speed of healing, and the motion of the hip, spine and leg. Another important goal is to shorten the time needed to return to activity and sport.

The intensity of the rehabilitation depends on whether the fracture was stable or unstable.

In people with surgical treatment, physical therapy starts after one or 2 days of bed rest. It is initiated with training of small movements, transfers, and exercise training. Active ankle foot and toes movements, active hip abduction both sides, static quadriceps exercises can start immediately after surgery and should be done at least four times a day, 10 times every hour.

Extension of the knee in sitting, once the patient can sit in a chair or wheelchair comfortably 10−15 times every hour.

During the nonweight bearing status, the patient performs isometric gluteal and quadriceps exercises, range of motion exercises, and upper-extremity resistive exercises. Once weight-bearing is resumed, physical therapy consists of gait training and resistive exercises for the trunk and extremities, along with endurance exercises such as treadmill or bicycle training. Stabilization exercises and mobility training should also be remained in the program. Hydrotherapy is also good and helpful when available.

Mobility training is useful to regain the range of motion in the hip, knee, and ankle after immobilization. Gait training should start with walking between parallel bars. Afterward the patient should learn how to walk with a walker or with a cane. Full weight bearing is usually allowed by 3 months—or when your bones are fully healed. Balance and proprioception training should also be included in the rehabilitation. Resistive training should be progressive to improve the muscle strength in the hip and leg. In the final stage functional exercises should be included to provide the patient with an optimal return of function.

In pelvic fractures in the elderly population, the rehabilitation process will be focused on optimizing their quality of life. Rapid mobilization and sufficient pain relief are the main objectives of treatment and appointment of the home to assess the need, for example, rails, ramps, increased lighting, removal of loose mats. Appropriate walking aids should also be supplied. A fall prevention outpatient program could be of benefit.

Zidén et al. investigated the long-term effect of a home rehabilitation program. They concluded that 1 year after the start of the rehabilitation process, most patients didn't consider themselves fully recovered, compared to their situation before the fracture [12]. There should be more investigations to describe the short-term and long-term effects of the rehabilitation for pelvic fractures.

Complications

Possible complications include

- Wound healing problems, including infection
- Damage to nerves or blood vessels
- Blood clots
- Pulmonary embolism—a blood clot in the lungs

Dislocation

Posterior dislocation is more than anterior. Hip joint is more stable in abduction, extension, internal rotation, and least stable in flexion, adduction. Femoral head is less supported by the acetabulum and more dependent on joint capsule for stability. Spontaneous dislocation of the hip by the strong pull of the spasmodic hip flexors and adductors may occur in painful arthritis or in case of spina bifida, PPRP, CP, etc. due to muscle imbalance.

Most common form of injury is dashboard injury in which the impact is transmitted through the bend knee which is closer to the dashboard. The person sitting with crossed leg in the front seat may develop posterior dislocation of hip joint. Collapse of the roof on stooping coalminers may result in dislocation. If the hip is not fully adducted, fracture dislocation occurs. Posterior lip of acetabulum may be driven backwards by the head of the femur. If the hip is not adducted at all, the falling of the roof on the back of stooping coalminers may result in central fracture dislocation and anterior dislocation may occur when the hips are widely abducted. Anterior hip dislocation occurs due to hitting by the car from behind. Anterior dislocation occurs due to head on collision while driving a bike. Anterior dislocation is of two types:

- **High**—the head of femur lies over the pelvic crest in marked internal rotation, full extension and some degree of abduction attitude. It is produced by forced external rotation, abduction in extension due to hitting by the car from the back of pedestrian.
- **Low**—anterior dislocation occurs by full extension, rotation, abduction in flexion due to head on collision of the bike. The head of the femur lies over the obturator foramen with 60° of abduction, full external rotation, and some degree of flexion

Incidence of posterior dislocation is more common than anterior with **20:1** ratio.

Clinical feature

There is shortening with adduction, internal rotation, and side flexion attitude. Femoral head may be palpated on buttock. One finds difficulty in palpating femoral pulse. No movement is possible.

Management

Reduce under anesthesia. The patient lying on the floor, fix the pelvis with the hip and knee flexed to 90°, pull the shaft of femur vertically upward and derotate. Sometimes it requires abduction to achieve reduction. Following reduction rest should be given for 3 weeks by traction/hip spica immobilization. During immobilization active ankle-foot-toe movement, static quadriceps, deep breathing exercise, bed mobility should be encouraged. After 3 weeks, encourage nonweight bearing hip movement and partial weight bearing walking with walking aids may be allowed. In case of associated fracture/myositis ossificans prolonged immobilization may be required.

Complications

1. **Fracture acetabulum**: The posterior rim of acetabulum may be fractured, which gets reduced during reduction of dislocation. Immobilization for 6 weeks and weight bearing is deferred for another 6 weeks. Large fracture fragment requires internal fixation and open reduction.

2. **Fracture head of femur**: A fragment of head of femur may get fractured by hitting against the posterior rim of acetabulum. Small fracture fragment usually gets reduced during reduction of dislocation. Relatively larger fragment, not correctly reduced may require excision. Following reduction 6 weeks immobilization and further 6 week no weight bearing should be given.

3. **Nerve injury**: Sciatic nerve that lies behind the hip joint may get injured in about 10%−13% of hip dislocation [13]. The incidence is three times more common in fracture dislocation than simple dislocation. Four out of five sciatic nerve injury is incomplete, involves the peroneal nerve, and recovers spontaneously. Damage by the fracture fragment may require surgery.

4. **Avascular Necrosis**: It is a late complication. The incidence is about 10% of dislocation due to thrombosis or damage to circumflex femoral arteries and artery accompanying ligamentum teres [14]. It leads to ischemic necrosis of head of femur and early secondary osteoarthritis.

5. **Myositis ossificans**: Occurs following repeated manipulation. Vigorous injury and repetitive manipulation increase the probability of myositis. To minimize/ avoid the risk of myositis rest should be given following manipulation by traction followed by hip spica.

6. **Irreducible dislocation**: Reduction becomes difficult by the presence of fracture fragment/soft tissue so it requires open reduction. Unreduced dislocation after a few weeks can't be reduced by closed method due to secondary soft tissue changes that prevent reduction it requires open reduction. Overtime articular cartilage gets degenerated and necrosis of the head of the femur may develop.

7. **Recurrent dislocation**: Every time hip is medially rotated it is displaced posteriorly/dislocate anteriorly from lateral rotation. Recurrent dislocation is often associated with fracture. A rent in gluteus minimus and posterior joint capsule also results in recurrent dislocation. It requires double bracing.

Management of anterior dislocation

Closed manipulative reduction is done under anesthesia. Subject in supine position fixes the pelvis with the hip and knee flexed. Pull the thigh upward and adduct the thigh to reduce the dislocation. Apply traction to maintain the reduction/hip spica immobilization with the hip in neutral position for 3 weeks. After 3 weeks the plaster/traction is removed and nonweight bearing walking with the help of walking aids can be initiated. In the absence of associated fracture/myositis ossificans partial weight bearing crutch gait can be started. In case of associated fracture and/or myositis ossificans another 3 weeks nonweight bearing should be given and partial weight bearing crutch gait starts after about 6 weeks.

Central dislocation

It is always associated with fracture acetabulum. It is of two types.

- **Intact weight bearing articular surface**—it results from blow upon the flexed knee so that the force transmitted through long axis of femur results in central dislocation. There will be shortening present.
- **Acetabulum is reduced to a back of bone**—it occurs from direct blow from site of GT at pelvis i.e., fall on the side/car hits the pedestrian while crossing the road. There occurs fracture of acetabulum floor and central dislocation.

Clinical feature

Sign of direct blow on GT, that is, bruising present and tenderness present over GT. There is no LLD, active movement painful, passive abduction, and internal rotation painful and limited. There may occur damage to genitourinary tract resulting in retention of urine. Damage to the greater vessels may lead to intrapelvis hemorrhage and shock.

Management

Depends on the degree of comminution and displacement. Usually managed conservatively by strong pull on the thigh and adduction.

The second type of injury can be managed by trochanteric traction. Following traction, the reduction is maintained by either tibial (type 1)/trochanteric (type 2) pin traction for 6 weeks.

In young persons with closed reduction not satisfactory, open reduction and large fragment is fixed by screw. Following open reduction, skeletal traction immobilization is given for 4–6 month. Open reduction is indicated in few cases of type 1 fracture dislocation and fix with screw/K wire fixation through posterior approach. Traction immobilization till wound heals followed by hip spica immobilization. During immobilization encourage active ankle-foot-toe movement, static quadriceps, gluteal exercise. After a few weeks, nonweight bearing movement without pain under traction can be given. Early nonweight bearing movements aid in molding/smoothening the acetabular articulating surface. Partial weight bearing is allowed after 8–10 weeks and full weight bearing after 12–14 days.

Complications

Urogenital damage, hemorrhage, damage to greater vessel, stiffness of hip joint, secondary OA may develop.

Avascular necrosis of the femoral head

Avascular necrosis, also called osteonecrosis or bone infarction, is a pathological condition affecting the femoral head in which there is death of bone tissue due to interruption of the blood supply. Essentially, the femoral head receives less blood supply. Since bone is living tissue when this blood supply is reduced enough the bone dies. Once the bone dies, the femoral head collapses and if severe enough, the hip joint itself collapses. AVN of the hip is poorly understood, but this process is the final common pathway of traumatic or nontraumatic factors that compromise the already precarious circulation of the femoral head. Femoral head ischemia results in the death of marrow and osteocytes and usually results in the collapse of the necrotic segment.

Causes

Avascular Necrosis mainly affects those aged between 20 and 50 years old. Males are more commonly affected than females.

It usually comes about secondary to an underlying health issue or previous injury. Avascular necrosis arises either as a result of traumatic or nontraumatic means. Sustaining a dislocated hip can result in a traumatic onset of avascular necrosis. Up to 20% of people, who dislocate their hip or fracture dislocation, develop avascular necrosis of the femoral head.

Nontraumatic avascular necrosis can arise from an array of issues, most notably excessive alcohol use, chronic corticosteroid use and blood clots/any damage to the arteries supplying the femur. The condition may also occur without any clear reason.

Avascular necrosis of the femoral head in children is known as Legg–Calvé–Perthes syndrome [15]. The main risk factors are alcoholism, fracture, fracture dislocation, and the use of high dose steroids [16]. Other risk factors include radiation therapy, chemotherapy, and organ transplantation. Osteonecrosis is also associated with cancer, lupus, sickle cell disease, HIV infection, Gaucher's disease, Caisson disease, diabetes, pancreatitis, autoimmune deficiencies/diseases, hypertension, vasculitis, etc.

Pathophysiology

The hematopoietic cells are most sensitive to low oxygen and are the first to die after reduction or cessation of the blood supply, usually within 12 h. Experimental evidence suggests that bone cells (osteocytes, osteoclasts, osteoblasts etc.) die within 12–48 h and that bone marrow fat cells die within 5 days.

Upon reperfusion, repair of bone occurs in 2 phases. First, there is angiogenesis and movement of undifferentiated mesenchymal cells from adjacent living bone tissue grow into the dead marrow spaces, as well as entry of macrophages that degrade dead cellular and fat debris. Second, there is cellular differentiation of mesenchymal cells into osteoblasts or fibroblasts. Under favorable conditions, the remaining inorganic mineral volume forms a framework for establishment of new, fully functional bone tissue.

The pathophysiology behind the association of chronic corticosteroid and alcohol use with avascular necrosis isn't fully understood but it is proposed that the overuse of the aforementioned substances interferes with the breakdown of fatty substances, which consequently deposited within the blood vessels. The narrow blood vessels interfere with blood supply to the femoral head. As the blood supply is reduced enough, the bone begins to undergo necrosis.

Signs and symptoms

Avascular necrosis requires time for its onset. It is relatively asymptomatic to begin, but as it progresses, gradually joint pain may develop which may limit the ability to move. Over time the pain becomes more pronounced. Pain limits both passive and active hip range of motion is the ultimate symptom, which can refer pain down the front of the thigh up to knee. Generally, the pain will arise when pressure is placed on the bone which unfortunately includes walking around.

Avascular necrosis can often mask itself as other conditions in the early phase given its general pain presentation within the hip. Therefore, it is paramount to record a detailed history of presentation and perform a thorough examination to diagnose avascular necrosis of head of femur.

Diagnosis

Diagnosis is typically by medical imaging such as X-ray, CT scan, or MRI. Rarely biopsy may be used.

X-ray images of avascular necrosis in the early stages usually appear normal. In later stages, it appears relatively more radio-opaque due to the nearby living bone becoming resorbed secondary to reactive hyperemia. The necrotic bone itself does not show increased radiographic opacity, as dead bone cannot undergo bone resorption which is carried out by living osteoclasts. Late radiographic signs also include a radiolucency area following the collapse of subchondral bone (crescent sign) and ringed regions of radiodensity resulting from saponification and calcification of marrow fat following medullary infarcts.

Other scans are less useful and are more specific to certain stages of the injury such as a bone scan or CT scan. The MRI can be used as a diagnostic tool and also as a means to monitor the remodeling/healing.

Treatment

Treatments may include medication, not walking on the affected leg, stretching, and surgery. Most of the time surgery is eventually required and may include core decompression, osteotomy, bone grafts, or joint replacement. The aim of conservative treatment is to decrease the weight bearing load through the head of the femur, usually by implementing crutches. To minimize loading over head of femur, reduce body weight in obese or overweight individuals and activities modifications is required. Avoid or minimize standing, whenever standing is required stand leaning against some support, stand with one leg forward and keep changing the leg positions. Loading the hip joint in extension minimizes load over the head of femur. To attain the congruent position, mobilize the hip joint to improve extension, internal rotation, and abduction range. Stretching of hip flexors, adductors are also important. Strengthening of glutei by static, thera-band resisted exercises help in deloading the hip joint. Auto-stretching should be taught to perform at home regularly.

Research has shown that the condition still progresses in 1−2 years. Without definitive treatment, 70%−80% of all avascular necrosis of the femoral head cases will progress and inevitably undergo surgery [17]. Irrespective of what surgery is undertaken, the primary goal is always to preserve the natural femoral head as opposed to replacing it.

There have been proposed nonoperative treatments that can be implemented before the condition progresses and the femoral head collapses. One of the most well-known and successful treatments, if the condition is identified early enough, is the core decompression i.e. decrease the pressure inside the femoral head. Internal bone pressure is relieved by drilling a hole into the bone, and a living bone chip and an electrical device to stimulate new vascular growth are implanted; and the free vascular fibular graft, in which a portion of the fibula, along with its blood supply, is removed and transplanted into the femoral head. This has proven to be successful, especially in those with early stages avascular necrosis based on preoperative and postoperative MRI studies.

Progression of the disease could possibly be halted by transplanting nucleated cells from bone marrow into avascular necrosis lesions after core decompression, although much further research is needed to establish this technique.

A variety of methods may be used to treat the most common being the total hip replacement (THR). However, THRs have a number of downsides including long recovery times and short life spans (of the hip joints). THRs are an effective means of treatment in the older population; however, in younger people they may wear out before the end of a person's life.

Other techniques such as metal on metal resurfacing may not be suitable in all cases of avascular necrosis; its suitability depends on how much damage has occurred to the femoral head. Bisphosphonates which reduce the rate of bone breakdown may prevent collapse due to AVN.

Prognosis

The amount of disability that results from avascular necrosis depends on what part of the bone is affected, how large an area is involved, and how effectively the bone rebuilds itself. The process of bone rebuilding takes place after an injury as well as during normal growth [18]. Normally, bone continuously breaks down and rebuilds—old bone is resorbed and replaced with new bone. The process keeps the skeleton strong and helps it to maintain a balance of minerals. In the course of avascular necrosis, however, the healing process is usually ineffective and the bone tissues break down faster than the body can repair them. If left untreated, the disease progresses, the bone collapses, and the joint surface breaks down, leading to pain and arthritis.

Hip labral tears

Hip labral tears are more common in people who play certain sports or who have structural abnormalities of the hip. Athletes who participate in sports such as ice hockey, soccer, football, golf and ballet are at higher risk of developing hip labral tears. Structural abnormalities of the hip also can lead to a hip labral tear.

Causes

The cause of a hip labral tear might be:

- **Trauma.** Injury to or dislocation of the hip joint—which can occur during car accidents or from playing contact sports such as football or hockey, soccer, and golf—can cause a hip labral tear.
- **Structural abnormalities.** Conditions that cause abnormal hip movement can also lead to hip labral tears. In femoroacetabular impingement (FAI), the femoral head doesn't fit into the socket properly. This imperfect fit can cause long-lasting groin pain and movement limitations. This is the most common cause of labral tears.
- **Repetitive motions.** Sports-related and other physical activities—including long-distance running and the sudden twisting or pivoting motions common in golf or softball—can lead to joint wear and tear that ultimately result in a hip labral tear.

Clinical features

Many hip labral tears cause no signs or symptoms. Some people, however, have one or more of the following:

- Pain in your hip or groin, often made worse by long periods of standing, sitting, or walking.
- A locking, clicking or catching sensation in your hip joint.
- Stiffness or limited range of motion in your hip joint.

The test is considered positive if one or more of these symptoms are reproduced during the test: click, clunk, or pain in the groin region.

- Impingement test—The hip joint is passively flexed to 90°, internally rotated, and adducted.
- FABER test—The lower extremity is passively placed in a figure-of—four position, and slight pressure is applied to the medial side of the knee.
- Resisted straight leg raise test—The patient's hip is flexed 30° with the knee in extension and a downward pressure applied.
- McCarthy sign/Thomas test (hip flexion to extension maneuver)—With the patient in a supine position, the subject fully flexes both hips. The examiner slowly/passively extends the subject's lower extremities and moves the hips into external rotation. The test is repeated, but with the hip in internal rotation.
- Internal rotation load/grind test—With the patient in a supine position, the examiner passively flexes the patient's hip to 100° and then rotates the subject's hip from internal rotation to external rotation while pushing along the axis of the femur through the knee to elicit "grind."
- Fitzgerald test—For assessment of the anterior labrum. The patient's hip is acutely flexed and then extended while internally rotated and in full abduction.
- Patrick test—For assessment of the posterior labrum. The patient's hip is flexed and then extended while in abduction and external rotation.

Imaging tests can also help doctors diagnose a hip labral tear. The doctor may order the following imaging tests:

- **X-rays**: X-rays can alert doctors to problems with the hip bones, such as FAI, or osteoarthritis, that may contribute to a labral tear and a painful hip.
- **Magnetic resonance imaging (MRI)**: This test shows more details in soft tissues. An MRI can show where a labral tear is, and how severe it is.

Complications—A hip labral tear can make you more likely to develop osteoarthritis in that joint in the future.

Prevention—If the sports you play put a lot of strain on your hips, condition the surrounding muscles with strength and flexibility exercises.

Physical therapy management—Movements that cause stress in the area need to be avoided. The rehabilitation protocol following acetabular labral debridement or repair is divided into four phases.

Phase 1—initial exercise (week 1—4)

The primary goals following an acetabular labral debridement or repair are to the minimize pain and the inflammation, and initiate early motion exercises. This phase initially consists of isometric contraction exercises for the hip adductors, abductors, transverse abdominals, and extensor muscles. Following a labral debridement, closed-chain activities such as low-level leg press or shuttle can begin with limited resistance.

Weight bearing protocol following a debridement is 50% for 7–10 days, and non-weight bearing or toe-touch weight bearing for 3–6 weeks in case of a labral repair. Unnecessary hypomobility will limit progress in future phases, thus it is important to ensure that the patient maintains adequate mobility and range during this phase.

Treatment modalities

- Aquatic therapy is a suitable treatment approach—movement in the water allows for improvement in gait by allowing appropriate loads to be placed on the joint without causing unnecessary stress to the healing tissue. For example, the patient may perform light jogging in the water using a flotation device. It is import to know that the patient's range of motion precautions, as these may vary in debridement or repair [19].
- Manual therapy for pain reduction and improvement in joint mobility and proprioception. Considerations include gentle hip joint mobilizations, contract-relax stretching for internal and external rotators, long axis distraction, and assessment of lumbo-sacral mobility.
- Cryotherapy.
- Appropriate pain management through medication.
- Gentle stretching of hip muscle groups including piriformis, psoas, quadriceps, hamstring muscles with passive range of motion.
- Stationary bike without resistance, with seat height that limits the hip to less than 90°.
- Exercises such as: water walking, piriformis stretch, ankle pumps.

To progress to phase 2, ROM has to be greater or equal to 75%.

Phase 2—intermediate exercise (week 5–7)

The goal of this phase is to continue to improve ROM and soft tissue flexibility. Manual therapy should continue with mobilization that is more aggressive, passive ROM exercises should become more aggressive as needed, for external and internal rotation.

- Flexibility exercises involving the piriformis, adductor group, psoas/rectus femoris should continue
- Stationary bike with resistance
- Side stepping with an abductor band for resistance
- Core strengthening such as bridging
- Noncompetitive swimming
- Exercises such as wall sits with abductor band, two leg bridging

To progress to the third phase, it is important that the patient has a normal gait pattern with no Trendelenburg sign. The patient should have symmetrical and passive ROM measurement with minimal complaints of pain [20].

Phase 3—advanced exercise (week 8–12)

- Manual therapy should be performed as needed.
- Flexibility and passive ROM interventions should become slightly more aggressive if the limitations persist (if the patient has reached his full ROM or flexibility, terminal stretches should be initiated).
- Strengthening exercises: walking lunges, lunges with trunk rotations, resist end sport cord, walking forward/backwards, plyometric bounding in the water.
- Exercises such as core ball stabilization, golf progression, lunges.

To progress to the fourth phase, it is important that there is symmetrical ROM and flexibility of the psoas and piriformis.

Phase 4—sport specific training (12 week onwards)

In this phase, it is important to return safely and effectively back to competition or previous activity level. Manual therapy, flexibility, and ROM exercises can continue as appropriate.

It is important the patient has good muscular endurance, good eccentric muscle control, and the ability to generate power.

The patient can be given sport specific exercises and has to have the ability to demonstrate a good neuromuscular control of the lower extremity during the activities.

Exercises such as sport specific drills and functional testing.

References

[1] Osterhoff G, Morgan EF, Shefelbine SJ, Karim L, McNamara LM, Augat P. Bone mechanical properties and changes with osteoporosis. Injury 2016;47(Suppl. 2):S11–20.

[2] Yoo H, Cho Y, Hwang S. Outcomes of combined neck and trochanter fractures of the femur treated with cephallomedullary nail in elderly. Hip Pelvis 2019;31(4):200–5.

[3] Raaymakers EL, Marti RK. Nonunion of the femoral neck: possibilities and limitations of the various treatment modalities. Indian J Orthop 2008;42(1):13–21.

[4] Attum B, Pilson H. Intertrochanteric femur fracture [Updated 2021 Aug 11]. In: StatPearls [Internet]. Treasure Island, FL: StatPearls Publishing; January 2022. Available from: https://www.ncbi.nlm.nih.gov/books/NBK493161/.

[5] Medda S, Reeves RA, Pilson H. Subtrochanteric femur fractures [Updated 2021 Aug 4]. In: StatPearls [Internet]. Treasure Island, FL: StatPearls Publishing; January 2022. Available from: https://www.ncbi.nlm.nih.gov/books/NBK507803/.

[6] Rizkalla JM, Nimmons SJB, Jones AL. Classifications in brief: the Russell-Taylor classification of subtrochanteric hip fracture. Clin Orthop Relat Res 2019;477(1):257–61.

[7] Lu Y, Uppal HS. Hip fractures: relevant anatomy, classification, and biomechanics of fracture and fixation. Geriatr Orthop Surg Rehabil 2019;10. 2151459319859139.

[8] Davis DD, Foris LA, Kane SM, et al. Pelvic fracture [Updated 2021 Nov 7]. In: Stat-Pearls [Internet]. Treasure Island, FL: StatPearls Publishing; January 2022. Available from: https://www.ncbi.nlm.nih.gov/books/NBK430734/.

[9] Furey AJ, O'Toole RV, Nascone JW, Sciadini MF, Copeland CE, Turen C. Classification of pelvic fractures: analysis of inter- and intraobserver variability using the Young-Burgess and Tile classification systems. Orthopedics 2009;32(6):401.

[10] Incagnoli P, et al. Early management of severe pelvic injury (first 24 hours). Anaesth Crit Care Pain Med 2019;38(2):199–207.

[11] Rommens PM, Hopf JC, Arand C, Handrich K, Boudissa M, Wagner D. Prospective assessment of key factors influencing treatment strategy and outcome of fragility fractures of the pelvis (FFP). Eur J Trauma Emerg Surg 2022. https://doi.org/10.1007/s00068-022-01887-1.

[12] Zidén L, Kreuter M, Frändin K. Long-term effects of home rehabilitation after hip fracture – 1-year follow-up of functioning, balance confidence, and health-related quality of life in elderly people. Disabil Rehabil 2010;32(1):18–32.

[13] Dawson-Amoah K, Raszewski J, Duplantier N, Waddell BS. Dislocation of the hip: a review of types, causes, and treatment. Ochsner J 2018;18(3):242–52.

[14] Kellam P, Ostrum RF. Systematic review and meta-analysis of avascular necrosis and posttraumatic arthritis after traumatic hip dislocation. J Orthop Trauma 2016;30(1):10–6.

[15] McCarthy RE. Avascular necrosis of the femoral head in children. Instr Course Lect 1988;37:59–65.

[16] Barney J, Piuzzi NS, Akhondi H. Femoral head avascular necrosis [Updated 2022 Jan 19]. In: StatPearls [Internet]. Treasure Island, FL: StatPearls Publishing; January 2022. Available from: https://www.ncbi.nlm.nih.gov/books/NBK546658/.

[17] Sen RK. Management of avascular necrosis of femoral head at pre-collapse stage. Indian J Orthop 2009;43(1):6–16.

[18] Matthews AH, Davis DD, Fish MJ, et al. Avascular necrosis [Updated 2021 Oct 9]. In: StatPearls [Internet]. Treasure Island, FL: StatPearls Publishing; January 2022. Available from: https://www.ncbi.nlm.nih.gov/books/NBK537007/.

[19] Torres-Ronda L, Del Alcázar XS. The properties of water and their applications for training. J Hum Kinet 2014;44(1):237–48.

[20] Gogu S, Gandbhir VN. Trendelenburg sign [Updated 2021 Nov 21]. In: StatPearls [Internet]. Treasure Island, FL: StatPearls Publishing; January 2022. Available from: https://www.ncbi.nlm.nih.gov/books/NBK555987/.

Overuse conditions

Trochanteric bursitis

One of the common causes of lateral hip pain is trochanteric bursitis. In case of Trochanteric Bursitis, two bursae are commonly involved: Subgluteus Medius bursa is located above the greater trochanter and underneath the insertion of the gluteus medius. Subgluteus Maximus bursa is located between the greater trochanter and the insertion of the gluteus medius and gluteus maximus muscles [1].

It is frequently seen in soccer players. Relatively rare condition, chronic trochanteric bursitis usually develops due to prolonged pressure over the bursa. The incidence is common between 4th and 5th decades of life. Acute traumatic trochanteric bursitis frequently occurs in young age group.

Superficial trochanteric bursa lies slightly anteriorly underneath gluteus minimus muscle, deep trochanteric bursa lies slightly posteriorly underneath gluteus medius muscle, and sub-gluteus maximus bursa lies lateral to the greater trochanter underneath gluteus maximus and tensor fascia lata fibres. It facilitates gliding of anterior portion of gluteus maximus tendon as it passes over the greater trochanter to inert into iliotibial band. Iliotibial band is a nonelastic dense collagenous band that is formed by condensation of fascia lata, deep fascia on the lateral aspect of thigh. It is attached from the iliac crest to lateral aspect of shaft of tibia about 4 cm below the joint line. Gluteus maximus is inserted to ITB from the posterior aspect, and tensor fascia lata is inserted to it from anterior aspect. Both the muscles work antagonist to each other to balance the pelvis. Gluteus maximus extends, lateral rotates the hip and tilts the pelvis backward, whereas tensor fascia lata causes flexion, abduction, and medial rotation of hip and tilts the pelvis forward. Hip flexion during the swing phase of gait cycle pulls the ITB anterior to greater trochanter and at midstance extension rubs across the bony prominence of the greater trochanter. Repetitive friction and microtrauma may give rise to chronic trochanteric bursitis.

Repetitive fall and blow in soccer players may cause microtrauma and adhesion formation due to chronic inflammation. Repetitive hip adduction while kicking the ball tense the ITB and compresses the underlying bursa against the greater trochanter predisposing to chronic trochanteric bursitis.

ITB tightness, imbalance between hip abductors and adductors muscle strength, pelvic tilt, leg length discrepancy, walking, or running in uneven ground, etc. are the predisposing factors that increase friction and chronic trochanteric bursitis.

Women are more likely to develop trochanteric bursitis. Women with wider pelvis have greater coxavara and genu valgus angulation. Greater prominence of greater trochanter stretches the ITB increasing friction [2].

Many time overpronation of the foot also causes it. As with overpronation, the knee falls inwards which increase the angle at the hip. Weakness in the hip abductors, especially gluteus medius has the same effect. Tight structures surrounding the hip such as the iliotibial band, hip flexors, and hamstrings also predispose to bursitis. A bone spur which is a small excess growth of bone can also aggravate the bursa.

Lying on the side compresses the trochanteric bursa, present underneath the gluteus maximus muscle over the greater trochanter. Lying on opposite side may also result in chronic bursitis due to adduction of the thigh and compression of the bursa by the tight IT band.

Occasionally acute trochanteric bursitis develops with particular activities such as getting out of a car during which a snap is felt at the lateral or posterolateral aspect of the hip region. Probably the tight IT band snaps over the trochanter mechanically irritating the bursa.

Clinical feature

Usually, gradual onset of pain on the lateral aspect of hip region may radiate over the L_5 segment [3]. One complains of lateral thigh pain up to the knee and occasionally felt on the lateral aspect of leg. It is often confused with radiating pain over lumbosacral spine as the pain pattern resembles that of L_5 spinal lesion. Pain is dull aching in nature. Pain aggravates on step climbing, standing up from a low chair due to strong contraction of gluteus maximus. Side lying, sitting crossed leg is uncomfortable. One may wake up in the night due to pain as it rolls on affected side. Hip external rotation and abduction increases the pain. Patient may walk with antalgic gait.

On physical examination shifting of pelvis away from affected side may be seen suggestive of IT band tightness, genu valgus may be present [4]. Slight limping may be present while walking. Active physiological movements are full and free. Passive abduction may cause pain at end range as the bursa gets squeezed between the GT and pelvis. Passive adduction may be limited suggestive of IT band tightness. Combined flexion, adduction, internal rotation may reproduce the pain as the bursa gets compressed underneath the stretched gluteus maximus muscle. Resisted abduction and extension may be painful as the bursa gets compressed under the gluteus maximus. Joint plays normal in amplitude and pain free. Neuromuscular evaluation shows no abnormality. On palpation tenderness present over posterior aspect of GT [5].

Management

Acute bursitis can be managed by cryotherapy, rest from precipitating activities. Phonophoresis with analgesics may help in resolution of inflammation.

The goal is resolution of chronic inflammation and prevents recurrence. Avoid/ minimize step climbing, sitting crossed-leg, side lying, etc.

To promote resolution of chronic inflammation, apply US/SWD. LASER is also found to be effective.

IT band and tensor fascia lata stretching and stretching of hip abductors, adductors, hamstrings by muscle energy techniques is beneficial. Low-resistance strengthening of gluteus maximus to prevent recurrence is important [3].

Iliotibial band friction syndrome (ITBFS)

Iliotibial friction syndrome is a repetitive stress injury caused by excessive friction anywhere along the course of ITB. ITB originates from iliac crest and inserts to Gerdy's tubercle on lateral aspect of shaft of tibia about 4 cm below the joint line. Gluteus maximus is inserted from posteriorly and tensor fascia late is inserted from anteriorly to ITB. Contraction of gluteus maximus extends and rotates the hip externally and extends the knee through ITB. Contraction of TFL abducts, flexes, and rotates the hip internally and extends the knee through ITB [4]. During swing and stance phases of gait, the iliotibial tract translates anterior and posterior with respect to both the hip and knee joint axes. As the hip moves from extension to flexion, the proximal iliotibial tract passes from behind the greater trochanter to in front of it. During knee extension, the distal iliotibial band passes from behind to in front of the lateral femoral epicondyle. The repetitive friction caused by a tight iliotibial tract rubbing over the bony prominence of the greater trochanter or lateral epicondyle may result in irritation and inflammation as snapping hip syndrome or runner's knee, respectively.

Irritation may occur due to tightness of ITB near its origin at greater trochanter or near its insertion at lateral epicondyle of femur. The intrinsic precipitating factors include prominent lateral epicondyle of femur, tight ITB, genu varum, foot pronation, etc. and extrinsic factors includes training errors in runners, excessive downhill running, running on hard surface, running with excessive lateral heel wear of the foot wear, etc. Although iliotibial friction syndrome is frequently seen in long-distance runners, it can occur in anybody engaged in repetitive knee flexion-extension like circuit training, cycling, weight lifting, jumping, etc. activities. ITB moves anterior to the axis of knee joint during extension at about 30° and posterior to the axis of knee joint during flexion at about 30° [6].The forward and backward movements of ITB irritate the lateral epicondyle of femur and repetitive friction over time results in chronic inflammation of ITB, the bursa underneath it or the periosteum of the lateral femoral epicondyle. During swing phase of gait cycle, hip flexion by TFL pulls the ITB anterior to greater trochanter and knee flexion sweeps the ITB posterior to lateral epicondyle of femur and then acts as knee flexor. Thus, swing phase is characterized by simultaneous tensing of ITB across the hip and knee joints. The ITB undergoes maximal tension as it proximally lies anterior to hip joint and distally lies posterior to knee joint. This position of ITB to both hip and knee joints is maintained until midstance phase of gait cycle during which the knee is close to full extension and hip begins to extends. At midstance, ITB undergoes reversal of action at both hip and knee joints as extensors and rub against greater trochanter and lateral epicondyle of femur [7].

Gluteus maximus is a powerful hip and trunk extensor that plays great role in step climbing, running activities, tensor fascia lata acts antagonistically to gluteus maximus. Pelvis is dynamically balanced by opposing forces of these two muscles. Tightness of tensor fascia lata tilts the pelvis down and forward, genu valgus, lateral tracking dysfunction of patella, etc.

Women with broader pelvis have greater coxavara and genu valgus. Therefore, ITB in females sustained greater stretch across the greater trochanter and more incidence of proximal pathology, that is, trochanteric bursitis than distal pathology, that is, ITB friction syndrome.

Prolonged internal rotation of tibia associated with abnormal foot pronation results in antero-medial traction of the ITB insertion so that it is subjected to repetitive friction across lateral epicondyle of femur during stance phase of gait cycle [8]. In contrast foot with restricted pronation due to cavus deformity will cause excessive external rotation and genu varum resulting in distraction of lateral collateral ligament and ITB. The ITB is pulled across the lateral epicondyle of femur and is subjected to repetitive friction.

Running or jogging in uneven of hilly ground results in foot pronation of higher side and supination of lower side. Overpronation foot on uphill side is associated with internal rotation and genu valgus, whereas that on downhill side is associated with external rotation and genu varum. Distraction of ITB across lateral femoral epicondyle and repetitive friction may lead to ITB friction syndrome.

In case of leg length discrepancy, the shorter side sustains stress with overpronation foot and that on longer side bears weight over cavus foot posture. The longer side is prone to develop trochanteric bursitis, and the shorter side is prone to develop IT band friction syndrome.

ITB shifts anteriorly during each down-stroke pedaling and posteriorly on upstroke pedaling while cycling. Repetitive anterior and posterior movements subject it to friction and irritation.

Clinical features

Diffuse pain experienced on lateral aspect of knee. Persons with more pain may walk with stiff knee gait to avoid knee flexion. Pain aggravates by running, typically appears on starting and disappears with warming up. Pain is worse in downhill running, running in uneven ground, step climbing, etc. Occasionally swelling may develop on lateral femoral epicondyle. Localized tenderness is present on lateral epicondyle of femur; but not over lateral collateral ligament, postero-lateral knee capsule, popliteal tendon, etc. Patient may not complain of pain during sprinting, waking, squatting, etc. Ober's test shows ITB and TFL tightness and Noble compression test may be positive [9].

Management

Avoid the precipitating activities for about 4—6 weeks as this chronic overuse condition takes prolong period for resolution. Phonophoresis with salicylate cream or 10% hydrocortisone may help in resolution of inflammation and pain [10]. Moist heat or any other heating modality may be applied before stretching of tight ITB and TFL.

To stretch the ITB, subject is in side lying position on the sound side with the hip and knee flexed to increase the base of support. Therapist stands behind and places one hand on the pelvis, with the other hand support the bend knee while the leg is supported by the forearm. Abduct and hyper abduct the thigh till the pelvis is leveled and fix it. Extend and adduct the thigh and extend the knee with adduction of leg to stretch the ITB.

To stretch the tensor fascia lata, subject is in side lying position on the sound side with the hip and knee flexed to increase the base of support. Therapist stands behind and places one hand on the pelvis, with the other hand support the bend knee while the leg is supported by the forearm. Abduct and hyper abduct the thigh till the pelvis is leveled and fix it. Extend and adduct the thigh to stretch the TFL. In standing with the sound leg crossed in front of the affected and move the pelvis forward and away from the affected side to extend and adduct the hip joint.

To prevent recurrence, correction of underlying cause by foot wear modification is recommended. Overpronated foot may be benefited by medial heel wedge [11], genu varum, and supinated foot posture may require lateral heel and sole rise foot wear. Soft foot wear is helpful. Change the foot wear in case of excessive worn out sole.

Muscle strain

The common strained muscles of the hip are hamstring, adductors, and rectus femoris. Chronic muscle strain that leads to over use of hip adductor is common. Acute strain of rectus femoris and hamstring is due to over stress. Depending on the severity, strain is classified into **three grades**. In **first degree** strain, a few fibers are damaged. The anatomical and functional integrity of muscle is still maintained. Resisted isometric contraction is painful but strong. In **second degree** strain, more fibers are damaged. The anatomical and functional integrity is affected, resisted isometric contraction quick and painful. In **third degree** strain, there occur complete rupture; a visible/palpable gap may be present. Resisted isometric contraction is painless and weak [12].

The management depends on the degree of strain and nature of the lesion. To prevent further damage, avoid precipitating activities. Muscle is vulnerable to reinjury for 5—7 days. Therefore, adequate care must be given to protect the injured muscle. In acute strain, give rest to the part in elevation and compressive bandage. Apply ice for 20—25 min, 5—6 times/day for 48—72 h. The acuteness subsides movements with discomfort but no pain can be initiated. Movements in cold hydrotherapy pool can be given followed by movement in warm hydro pool. Apply US followed by DTFM, then passive stretching with discomfort but no pain. Encourage active movement to restore and maintain the gliding mechanism. Restore or maintain the muscle strength. After about 3 weeks, progressive stretching and strengthening exercises can be initiated. Vigorous stretching and strengthening can be given after 6 weeks. Following stretching and strengthening apply ice therapy.

In case of chronic tendinitis, avoid precipitating activities. Apply US/LASER followed by DTFM and passive stretching. Encourage active movements to restore the gliding mechanism and muscle strength.

Adductors strain

Adductors strain is also known as groin pull. It includes adductor longus, adductor magnus, adductor brevis, and pectineus muscles. Most commonly, adductor longus is affected (62.90%) [13]. Functions of adductors include stabilization of pelvis and lower extremity during stance phase of gait cycle. Adductors strain develops due to repetitive hip adductions as in soccer or repetitive hip abduction of hip joint as in skating, cross-country skiing, etc. Acute traumatic lesion occurs due to forceful stretching while the muscle works concentrically. Combined hip abduction and external rotation exerts eccentric tension and may result in strain. It may occur due to sudden change in direction or sudden acceleration while sprinting or running. Excessive abduction-external rotation of hip while kicking ball may cause over stretching of adductors and acute strain. Sustain use of hip adductors as in horse riders may also predispose to chronic strain. Therefore, adductors strain is also known as rider's strain. The predisposing factors are weak adductors, and reduced extensibility and bio-mechanical factors include leg length discrepancy and excessive foot pronation. The dominant leg is frequently involved.

One complains of acute onset groin pain following injury. Nature of pain is stabbing type. Since the attachment site adductor tendons is poor in vascularity and richly supplied by nerve endings, one complains of severe pain. Swelling and bruising develops slowly over time. Pain aggravates with activities. Tenderness present over the groin may be in the distal insertion of the muscle. Resisted hip adduction and passive stretching reproduce the symptoms. Complete rupture is characterized by the absence of muscle contraction.

Chronic over use injury is characterized by vague and diffuse pain in the groin, and pain may spread distally along the medial aspect of thigh or proximally toward the rectus abdominis [14]. Morning pain and stiffness, pain during exercise, stiffness after a period of rest are the characteristics. X-rays AP view of pelvis and frog leg view of affected hip may be considered to exclude avulsion injury, osteitis pubis, or stress fracture.

Management

Rest and ice compression for 20 min, 5–6 times per day is applied initially for 2–3 days. After about 2–3 days use ultrasound or phonophoresis, Cyriax's deep transverse friction massage and slow passive stretching with discomfort but no pain. Once full range of hip abduction without pain is achieved, and progressive strengthening of hip adductors can be initiated. Swimming is useful to improve endurance.

Pulled hamstrings injury

Pulled hamstring injury involves one of the three or more hamstrings. Injury occurs either due to overstretching or overloading. Incidence is more common in sprinters, long-distance runners, soccer players, racquet game, long jump, etc. Violent eccentric work of the muscle or forceful stretch may cause injury. Injury usually occurs during the last part of swing phase. The predisposing factors include weak hamstring strength, loss of flexibility, lack of warm-up, previous history of injury, fatigue— most hamstrings injury in football players occur in second half of the game, etc.

Audible snapping sound may be present at the time of injury with severe sharp pain on the back of the thigh and the victim falls down. Swelling develops within a few hours following injury and ecchymosis develops within 48 h [15]. Patient finds difficulty in extending the knee completely. Passive stretching and resisted knee flexion is painful.

Management

Grade 1 strain may feel like a tightness that heals within a few days. Moderate to severe strain requires treatment. Rest and ice compression 20–25 min, 5–6 times per day is applied for 72 h. After 72 h, ultrasound or phonophoresis with antiinflammatory analgesic cream with or without steroid is followed by gentle stretching with little discomfort. Hold and relax or muscle energy technique may be used to stretch the hamstrings. One can perform active straight leg raise as the pain allows. Once full knee extension without pain is achieved, progressive strengthening exercise can be initiated. Multiangle static hamstring exercises, eccentric hamstrings exercise by lowering the bend knee in prone lying can be given.

Running program starts when there is no pain, no swelling, full range of motion, and hamstrings strength is about 70% of sound side. One can return back to activities once the muscle strength becomes 80% of the sound side.

Rectus femoris strain

Rectus femoris injury occurs at its origin or upper third of the muscle [16]. Injury occurs due to vigorous hip flexion for sudden fast running start, football tackle, forced hip flexion against resistance, combined hip extension, and knee flexion, etc.

Patient experiences snapping sound with sudden stabbing pain in the anterior groin. Ecchymosis appears after about 48 h. Swelling, warmth, tenderness, localized firmness, etc. may be present. Passive knee flexion and resisted knee extension may be painful.

Management

Rest and ice compression 20−25 min, 5−6 times per day is applied for 72 h. After 72 h, ultrasound or phonophoresis with antiinflammatory analgesic cream with or without steroid is followed by gentle stretching with little discomfort. Static quadriceps exercise should be encouraged from the first day onwards. Strengthening program starts when there is no swelling, no pain, and full range of motion is present. Progressive strengthening is followed by eccentric activities. Quadriceps works concentrically during backward walking and running, and eccentrically during forward walking and running.

Osteitis pubis

First described in 1924, osteitis pubis has been known as a noninfectious inflammation of the pubis symphysis causing varying degrees of lower abdominal and pelvic pain [17]. Osteitis pubis was first described in patients who had undergone suprapubic surgery, and it remains a well-known complication of invasive procedures about the pelvis. It may also occur as an inflammatory process in athletes.

- **Causes**: Pregnancy and childbirth, gynecologic surgery, urologic surgery.
- Athletic activities such as running, football, soccer, ice hockey, tennis, etc.,
- Major trauma, repeated minor trauma,
- Rheumatological disorders,
- Overload or training errors, exercising on hard surfaces like concrete, exercising on uneven ground, beginning an exercise program after a long lay-off period, increasing exercise intensity or duration too quickly exercising in worn out or ill-fitting shoes.
- Biomechanical inefficiencies like faulty foot and body mechanics and gait disturbances, poor running or walking mechanics, tight and stiff muscles in the hips, groin, and buttocks, muscular imbalances, leg length differences.
- Unknown etiologies.

Pathomechanics: The symphysis pubis is a fibrocartilaginous joint between the pubic rami. In addition, the abdominal muscles (rectus abdominis and external and internal oblique muscles) attach distally to the inguinal ligament, conjoined tendon, and pubic symphysis, whereas the adductor muscles (pectineus, adductor longus, adductor brevis, adductor magnus, gracilis) arise from the superior and inferior rami of the pubis. The obturator and femoral nerves with their cutaneous branches have been suggested as etiologic factors in groin pain. Thus, dysfunctions that affect the pubic symphysis can affect either joint mobility or the musculotendinous attachments of the abdominal or adductor muscles. Muscle imbalances between the abdominal and hip adductor muscles have been suggested as an etiologic factor in osteitis pubis. Because of their attachments to the thoracic cage proximally and the pubis distally, the abdominal muscles act synergistically with the posterior paravertebral muscles to stabilize the symphysis, allowing single-leg stance while maintaining balance and contributing to the power and precision of the kicking leg. The adductors, because they stabilize the symphysis by bringing the lower extremity closer to the pelvis, are antagonists to the abdominal muscles. In addition, the adductor muscle group transmits mechanical traction forces toward the symphysis pubis during its activity as a prime mover in the soccer push pass, tackling, and directing the soccer ball. Imbalances between abdominal and adductor muscle groups disrupt the equilibrium of forces around the symphysis pubis, predisposing the athlete to a subacute periostitis caused by chronic microtrauma. This microtrauma exceeds the dynamic capacity of tissue for hypertrophic remodeling, resulting in tissue degeneration. Shear stress at the symphysis pubis can also cause sacroiliac dysfunction in osteitis pubis if hip internal rotation is limited in either flexion or extension. This shear stress is transmitted to the symphysis pubis, resulting in either antero-posterior movement of one half of the pelvis in relationship to the other in extension or proximal-distal movement in flexion.

Pregnancy: Damage can occur to the ligaments surrounding and bridging the pubic joint (symphysis) as a result of the hormone relaxin, which is secreted around the time of birth to soften the pelvic ligaments for labor. At this time, repetitive stress of falling, tripping, and slipping can injure ligaments more easily. The hormone usually disappears after childbirth, and the ligaments become strong again. In some women the weakness persists, and activities such as carrying their baby or stepping up even a small step can cause a slight but continuous separation or shearing in the ligaments of the symphysis where they attach to the joint surfaces, even causing lesions in the fibrocartilage and pubic bones. Symptoms include one or more of the following: pain in the pubic area, hips, lower back, and thighs. This can take months (or even years) to go away.

Symptoms: The symptoms of osteitis pubis can include loss of flexibility in the groin region, dull aching pain in the groin and lower abdominal region, or in more severe cases, a sharp stabbing pain when running, kicking, changing directions, or even during routine activities such as standing up or getting out of a car. Tenderness on palpation is also commonly present in the adductor longus origin. Aggravating activities include running, stepping, jumping, and kicking.

The athlete will often report an insidious onset of groin pain with no major traumatic incident.

Management: Manual techniques to restore full range of motion in the lumbar, sacral, and hip joints. Treatment includes soft tissue mobilization and manipulative techniques, muscle energy techniques for relaxation and lengthening of tight muscles, core control exercises (pelvic floor training), adductor strengthening by gentle isometric and resisted isotonic strengthening, gluteal strengthening, and stationary cycling.

Return to running program and graduated and progressive return to play.

Ultrasound was not applied to athletes younger than 18 years because of concern for damage to the epiphyseal plates; alternatively, they received electric stimulation treatment.

References

[1] Pumarejo Gomez L, Childress JM. Greater trochanteric syndrome [Updated 2021 Jul 25]. In: StatPearls [Internet]. Treasure Island, FL: StatPearls Publishing; January 2022. Available from: https://www.ncbi.nlm.nih.gov/books/NBK557433/.

[2] Hadeed A, Tapscott DC. Iliotibial band friction syndrome [Updated 2021 Dec 11]. In: StatPearls [Internet]. Treasure Island, FL: StatPearls Publishing; January 2022. Available from: https://www.ncbi.nlm.nih.gov/books/NBK542185/.

[3] Seidman AJ, Varacallo M. Trochanteric bursitis [Updated 2022 Feb 12]. In: StatPearls [Internet]. Treasure Island, FL: StatPearls Publishing; January 2022. Available from: https://www.ncbi.nlm.nih.gov/books/NBK538503/.

[4] Trammell AP, Nahian A, Pilson H. Anatomy, bony pelvis and lower limb, tensor Fasciae latae muscle [Updated 2021 Aug 13]. In: StatPearls [Internet]. Treasure Island, FL: StatPearls Publishing; January 2022. Available from: https://www.ncbi.nlm.nih.gov/books/NBK499870/.

[5] Le DT, Shah S. Greater trochanteric bursitis injection [Updated 2022 Jan 6]. In: StatPearls [Internet]. Treasure Island, FL: StatPearls Publishing; January 2022. Available from: https://www.ncbi.nlm.nih.gov/books/NBK573083/.

[6] Fairclough J, Hayashi K, Toumi H, Lyons K, Bydder G, Phillips N, Best TM, Benjamin M. The functional anatomy of the iliotibial band during flexion and extension of the knee: implications for understanding iliotibial band syndrome. J Anat 2006; 208(3):309−16.

[7] Hyland S, Graefe S, Varacallo M. Anatomy, bony pelvis and lower limb, iliotibial band (tract). In: StatPearls. Treasure Island, FL: StatPearls Publishing; 2022. PMID: 30725782.

[8] Seijas R, Sallent A, Galán M, Alvarez-Diaz P, Ares O, Cugat R. Iliotibial band syndrome following hip arthroscopy: an unreported complication. Indian J Orthop 2016; 50(5):486−91.

[9] Hutchinson LA, Lichtwark GA, Willy RW, Kelly LA. The iliotibial band: a complex structure with versatile functions. Sports Med 2022;52. https://doi.org/10.1007/s40279-021-01634-3.

[10] Hahn C. Applications of iontophoresis and phonophoresis. Phys Ther Schol Proj 1996; 185. https://commons.und.edu/pt-grad/185.

[11] Hemmati F, Forghany S, Nester C. The effects of pronated foot posture and medial heel and forefoot wedge orthoses on static balance in older people. J Foot Ankle Res 2014; 7(Suppl. 1):A17.

[12] Hayes KW, Petersen CM. Reliability of classifications derived from cyriax's resisted testing in subjects with painful shoulders and knees. J Orthop Sports Phys Ther 2003;33(5):235—46.

[13] Kiel J, Kaiser K. Adductor strain [Updated 2021 Jul 25]. In: StatPearls [Internet]. Treasure Island, FL: StatPearls Publishing; January 2022. Available from: https://www.ncbi.nlm.nih.gov/books/NBK493166/.

[14] Zini R, Volpi P, Bisciotti GN. Groin pain syndrome: a multidisciplinary guide to diagnosis and treatment. 1st ed. Cham, Switzerland: Springer; 2017.

[15] Karen JK, Hale EK, Geronemus RG. A simple solution to the common problem of ecchymosis. Arch Dermatol 2010;146(1):94—5.

[16] Kary JM. Diagnosis and management of quadriceps strains and contusions. Curr Rev Musculoskelet Med 2010;3(1—4):26—31.

[17] Gomella P, Mufarrij P. Osteitis pubis: a rare cause of suprapubic pain. Rev Urol 2017; 9(3):156—63. https://doi.org/10.3909/riu0767.

Further reading

[1] Lavine R. Iliotibial band friction syndrome. Curr Rev Musculoskelet Med 2010;3(1—4): 18—22.

Surgical conditions

Hip arthroplasty

Total hip replacement (THR) involves surgically removing the arthritic parts of the joint (cartilage and bone) replacing the "ball and socket" part of the joint with artificial components made from metal alloys and placing high-performance bearing surface between the metal parts. Most commonly the bearing surface is made from a very durable polyethylene plastic but other materials (including ceramics newer plastics or metals) have been used. Patients typically spend a few days in the hospital after the procedure (3–5 days are most typical) and some patients benefit from a short inpatient stay in a rehabilitation facility after that to help transition back to living independently at home. Most patients will walk with a walker or crutches for 3 weeks and then use a cane for another 4 weeks; after that the large majority of patients are able to walk freely.

A bewildering number of different implant designs bearing surface materials and surgical approaches have been tried to achieve one seemingly straightforward goal: improving the quality of life for patients who have hip arthritis. As with any important life decision, it makes good sense to get educated on those issues as they pertain to your hip.

The purpose of this article is to outline the essentials from a patient's perspective: who should think about having THR done what questions should a prospective patient ask the doctor and why one surgical approach or type of THR implant might be good for one patient but not for another.

Surgical options: bearing surfaces (polyethylene metal or ceramic)?

All hip replacements share one thing in common: they include a ball-and-socket joint. Materials which are used in the ball and in the socket togetherly is known as "bearing," like a bearing in a carhas the potential to affect the long-term durability of the joint replacement.

This is another area where technology may radically change the outcome of an operation; depending on how the research goes in this area hip replacement may look very different in 10 years than it does today. Or it may not.

Physiotherapy for the Hip Joint. https://doi.org/10.1016/B978-0-323-93649-1.00006-5

Many bearing surfaces have been tried in the 40 or 50 years that hip replacements have been done. And many more have failed than succeeded. That is one reason to proceed with caution given that we now have a bearing surface (metal-on-polyethylene) that has a track record going back to the 1960s.

Polyethylene is a durable high-performance plastic resin. It is slippery (which is why it does well in a mobile joint like the hip) but it is known to wear out. In fact, while more than 90% of metal-on-polyethylene bearing hip replacements (this is the most common bearing in use today) will be in service in 10 years many of those will not last 20 years [1]. And when the plastic wears out, it sometimes results in a destructive reaction causing bone loss around the joint. This can make repeat hip replacements (called revisions) more difficult.

Many types of plastics have been used in total hips but only one (ultrahigh-molecular-weight polyethylene) has stood the test of time. Teflon (like the nonstick material used in frying pans) was tried and abandoned because of severe reactions by surrounding tissue. Other modifications of polyethylene have been tried (including carbon-reinforced plastic) and abandoned because of durability problems. In fact, there is a new type of polyethylene gaining wide use today called highly cross-linked polyethylene which shows promising results in the lab but little if any data are available in people.

Ceramic bearing surfaces are sometimes used. These have been more popular in Europe than they have been in the United States. They may result in less aggressive wear but it is not known whether the wear they do cause will be more or less of a problem than wear from the traditional plastic bearings. Also fractures of ceramic bearings have been reported; as a result, some of these bearings have been taken out of service at the direction of the FDA.

Finally, metal-on-metal bearings have become popular. Interestingly they were tried early on in the history of hip replacement but problems related to their manufacture led to surgeons moving on to other designs. Now those problems have been overcome and they offer the potential to reduce bearing wear to almost immeasurable amounts. Some scientists question whether these devices will lead to increased amounts of metal ions or corrosive products being released in the body but to date these concerns have not been proved to be serious. However, because the renewed interest in these designs is fairly recent, there is comparatively little follow-up published in scientific journals about the longevity of hip replacements using metal-on-metal bearing surfaces.

The choice of which bearing to use is still somewhat controversial and reasonable scientists surgeons and patients will sometimes disagree. This is one of the most exciting areas of research in the field of hip replacement surgery. But as with surgical approach, it is worth considering the high likelihood of long-term success using traditional metal-on-polyethylene bearings when deciding whether to try another design that does not have results published beyond 10 years.

Surgical options: hemiresurfacing hip arthroplasty

This is a technique that can be used for some patients with avascular necrosis (also called osteonecrosis) of the femoral head. As mentioned previously that it is an arthritis-like condition of the hip; it may also affect the shoulders, knees or ankles. It is caused by an interruption of the blood circulation to the ball (the femoral head) of the ball-and-socket hip joint. This may be caused by trauma to the hip, excessive alcohol consumption, use of medical steroids like prednisone or any of numerous disorders of blood clotting.

When avascular necrosis is allowed to run its course, the result is usually severe degenerative joint disease and the treatment is usually traditional total hip replacement. Sometimes when the disease is caught early a joint-preserving procedure may be performed such as osteotomy (see below) core decompression or bone grafting.

In an intermediate stage of the disease avascular necrosis affects only the ball and not the socket; sometimes the top of the ball collapses resulting in a loss of roundness and this causes pain. At this stage, a resurfacing hip replacement may be an option. This involves putting a round metal "cap" on the ball and keeping the patient's own socket.

Advantages of this include the fact that it does not take away much bone (perhaps leaving more options available for subsequent reoperations) and that it is reasonably durable. Two studies have found that between 60% and 70% of these devices remain in service 10 years after the surgery [2]. This doesn't sound great compared to total hip replacement which has more than 90% success at that same time period but one must remember that patients with this stage of avascular necrosis are often quite young, that is, between 20 and 40 so total hip replacement is not considered an ideal approach for them.

The main disadvantage to this procedure apart from the failure rate is that pain relief is somewhat less than with traditional total hip replacement perhaps 80% as good, so many of these patients are left with some discomfort even after the surgery although most patients feel much better with the hemiresurfacing arthroplasty than they did before.

Patients with avascular necrosis have a complex set of choices to make and so it is best for them to find a surgeon who is extremely comfortable and experienced with a wide array of options to treat the painful hip.

Surgical options: pelvic osteotomy and hip fusion

Osteotomy is a procedure in which the bone around the socket of the hip joint is surgically cut so that the socket itself can be reoriented. This is best suited for young people with relatively early stages of arthritis particularly if the arthritis was caused by a childhood hip condition called developmental dysplasia of the hip.

Hip fusion is an operation that was more popular in the days before hip replacements were widely performed. This consists of surgically attaching the femur (thigh bone) to the pelvis and causing the two bones to heal together to become one. It results in loss of motion at the hip joint which is obviously a disadvantage but it is very reliable at relieving pain. It is seldom done anymore because most patients prefer to maintain motion about the hip but in the right circumstances it can still be a good choice. Patients who are otherwise poor candidates for hip replacement such as young people who plan to continue doing heavy manual laborer for a living or young patients with prior hip joint infections may decide that hip fusion is right for them.

Effectiveness

Current evidence suggests that traditional total hip replacements last more than 10 years in more than 90% of patients [3]. More than 90% of patients report having either no pain or pain that is manageable with use of occasional over-the-counter medications. The large majority of hip replacement patients are able to walk unassisted (i.e., without use of a cane) without any limp for reasonably long distances. Many have no distance restrictions at all and resume hiking golfing bicycling and other nonimpact recreational activities.

As mentioned, there are no studies to date documenting the short-term or long-term effectiveness of minimally invasive hip replacement and there are no studies that have proved that the joint replacement components can be reliably inserted with equal success or safety through the smaller incision used in minimally invasive hip replacement techniques.

In the event that a total hip replacement requires reoperation sometime in the future the results are generally good although often not as good as one typically gets with an uncomplicated first-time hip replacement. The results of repeat hip replacements (called "revisions") often depend on a number of factors that are not in the surgeon's (or the patient's) control such as infection, bone loss and condition of the muscles and other soft tissues around the hip joint. But in general, revision hip replacement can achieve a durable result and provide substantial relief of pain.

There is good evidence that the experience of the surgeon correlates with outcome in all kinds of joint replacements including total hip replacements. It is important that the surgeon performing the technique be not just a good general orthopedic surgeon but an expert experienced total hip replacement surgeon as well. It is reasonable to ask a surgeon whether (s)he concentrates his/her practice on joint replacements or whether (s)he does all kinds of orthopedic surgery.

Urgency

Total hip replacement for arthritis is elective surgery. With few exceptions, it does not need to be done urgently and can be scheduled around your other important life events.

Risks

Like any major surgical procedures total hip replacement is associated with certain medical and surgical risks. Although major complications are uncommon, they may occur. The possibilities include infection blood clots bleeding or blood transfusion and anesthesia-related or medical risks. Certain hip-specific risks like infection at the surgical site (typically less than 1.5%) dislocation (where the ball comes out of joint; less than 1% with one popular surgical technique) or other problems may also occur. However, the overall frequency of major complications following total hip replacement is low typically less than 5% (one in 20) depending on the individual's medical risk factors.

Later risks include the possibility that the device may loosen from the bone; late infections and dislocations may also occur. But again, numerous studies have shown that a technically well-performed total hip replacement is more than 90% likely to be in service and functioning well more than 10 years after the surgery.

Managing risk

Most of the major risks of total hip replacement can be treated. Use antibiotics before during and after surgery to minimize the likelihood of infection. They will take steps to decrease the likelihood of blood clots such as early patient mobilization and use of blood-thinning medications in some patients. Patients are evaluated by a good internist and/or anesthesiologist in advance of the surgery in order to decrease the likelihood of a medical or anesthesia-related complication. Great care is taken to be certain that the technical elements of the operation that are so important to success are correctly performed.

Again, the overall likelihood of a severe complication is generally less than 5% when such steps are taken.

Preparation

Patients undergoing a total hip replacement usually will undergo a preoperative surgical risk assessment by medicine physician and anesthesiologist in advance of the surgery. Routine blood tests are performed on all preoperative patients; chest X-rays and electrocardiograms are obtained in patients who meet certain age and health criteria as well. Surgeons and therapist should time with the patient in advance of the surgery making certain that all the patient's questions and concerns as well as those of the family are answered.

Timing

Total hip replacement for arthritis is elective surgery.

Next a well-positioned incision is made down the side of the hip. As already discussed, the location and length of the incision varies widely by approach and based on the patient's own anatomy.

Deeper tissues (muscles and tendons) are either spread or incised and prepared for later repair. The hip capsule (a thick covering directly on top of the ball and socket joint) is then opened. The ball is gently levered out of the socket and the arthritic ball is removed using a saw.

At this point, the damaged arthritic cartilage on the socket is removed using a scraping tool called a reamer and the socket (which may be misshapen from arthritis) is shaped to form a hemisphere. An artificial socket (called the acetabular component) is now inserted usually without using bone cement. Sometimes additional screws are used to hold the component firmly to the bone during the critical weeks following surgery when the patient's bone will attach itself to the metal on the artificial socket.

Next the inside of the thigh bone (femur) is prepared using motorized and hand-held tools to shape it to accept a stem at one end of which is the new artificial ball called the femoral head. Once the stem is inserted, leg length and joint stability are verified and the final components are inserted.

The tissues are cleaned with sterile saline solution (liquid) any deep tissues that were incised are now repaired and the skin is closed. A surgical drain may be used at the surgeon's decision.

Anesthetic

As mentioned, total hip replacement may be performed under epidural, spinal or general anesthesia. The choice is made in consultation with the surgeon and anesthesia provider.

Hospital stay

The average hospital stay is 3 days in length after a total hip replacement.

Recovery and rehabilitation in the hospital

Physical therapy is started on the day of (or the day after) surgery. Patients generally are encouraged to walk and to bear as much weight on the leg as they are comfortable doing. Other exercises to help with balance and getting into and out of bed are initiated on the day of surgery or the next morning.

Hospital discharge

Patients are encouraged to walk using a walker, crutches or cane as needed. Immediate weight bearing is permitted in most cases depending on other surgical circumstances.

Patients are allowed to walk following hospital discharge provided that there is no drainage coming from the incision site. On average patients are able to drive between two and 4 weeks after the surgery.

Each patient will be instructed for "Hip Precautions" after surgery. This is a short list of restrictions on particular motions designed to prevent dislocation of the joint replacement. Which specific precautions are used in an individual case depends on the approach used but in general patients are encouraged to avoid hip rotation and flexion. Low chairs, low couches and swivel chairs should be avoided. After about 6 weeks, some of those restrictions are relaxed, for example, most patients can easily put on shoes and socks once they've recovered from surgery and the surgeon gives them the OK but others including extreme flexion and rotation should always be limited to be on the safe side.

Physical therapy

Following hospital discharge, patients who undergo total hip replacement will participate in either home physical therapy or outpatient physical therapy to a location close to home.

Depending on the surgical approach used that therapy can begin right after discharge or it will start at 6 weeks after the surgery (the time when tissue healing of an important tendon has taken place). The surgeon will help you make the necessary arrangements.

The length of physical therapy varies based on patient age fitness and level of motivation but usually lasts about a month. Two to three therapy sessions per week are average for this procedure.

The specific therapy procedures vary with surgical approach but balance safe walking and reviewing hip precautions are emphasized early and muscle strengthening are goals later on.

Can rehabilitation be done at home?

As mentioned, this depends on each patient's individual circumstances. Age fitness level and having adequate help around the house are some of the elements that guide the choice.

All patients are given a set of home exercises to do between supervised physical therapy sessions and the home exercises make up an important part of the recovery process. However, supervised therapy which is best done in an outpatient physical therapy studio is extremely helpful and those patients who are able to attend outpatient therapy at the appropriate times after hospital discharge are encouraged to do so.

For patients who are unable to attend outpatient physical therapy, home physical therapy is arranged.

Usual response

On average patients walk with a walker or a pair of crutches for about 3 weeks then a cane for another month or so. The large majority of patients are able to walk without a limp and to resume reasonable personal and recreational activities gradually in the weeks and months following surgery.

The deep pain from the arthritis is usually noticeably absent right after surgery; the postoperative pain gradually improves and most patients have quit taking analgesics by about a month after surgery.

Returning to ordinary daily activities

The goal of total hip replacement is to return patients to a good level of function without hip pain. The large majority of patients are able to achieve this goal.

However, since the joint replacement components have no capacity to heal damage from injury sustained after surgery, some common-sense guidelines for athletic leisure and workplace activities are recommended as follows:

Recommended: Sedentary occupations (desk work), Cycling or stationary bike, Swimming, Water aerobics, cross-country skiing or Nordic Track, Golf.

Permitted: dancing, hiking, gentle doubles tennis, light labor (jobs that involve driving walking or standing but not heavy lifting).

Not recommended: jogging/running, impact exercises, sports that require twisting/pivoting (aggressive tennis basketball racquetball), contact sports, and Heavy labor.

Since the joint replacement includes a bearing surface which potentially can wear walking or running for fitness are not recommended. Patients generally feel well enough to do this and so need to exercise judgment in order to prolong the life-span of the implant materials. Swimming, water exercises, cycling, and cross-country skiing (and machines simulating it like Nordic Track) can provide a high level of cardiovascular and muscular fitness without excessive wear on the prosthetic joint materials.

As mentioned, certain precautions should be maintained for life in order to minimize the likelihood of dislocating the ball from the socket. Avoiding extreme twisting and bending from the hip are the most important of these.

Summary of total hip arthroplasty, hip resurfacing, and minimally invasive hip surgery for hip arthritis

Total hip replacement is a reliable operation in which the arthritic portions of a hip joint can be replaced with an artificial bearing surface. Pain is substantially improved and function regained in more than 90% of patients who have the operation [4].

Like any major procedure, there are risks to total hip surgery and the decision to have a hip replacement must be considered a quality-of-life choice that individual patients make with a good understanding of what those risks are.

Hip replacement is a surgical technique that has many variables; like most areas of medicine ongoing research will continue to help the technique evolve. It is important to learn as much as possible about the condition and the treatment options that are available before deciding whether—or how—to have a hip replacement done. While many of the changes now being explored in the field of total hip replacement may eventually be shown to be legitimate advances—perhaps including so-called minimally invasive surgical techniques as well as alternative bearing surfaces—it is important to compare them carefully to traditional total hip replacement performed using well established techniques which we know are 90%—95% likely to provide pain relief and good function for more than 10 years after the surgery.

Arthroplasty

It is a surgical procedure in which a painless, movable functional joint is reconstructed. It is two types:

- Excision Arthroplasty
- Replacement Arthroplasty

    Replacement arthroplasty is of two types:

- Hemi-arthroplasty
- Total hip replacement arthroplasty

Excision arthroplasty

It is a salvage procedure. It is performed when replacement arthroplasty fails. The head and neck of femur is excised, and the soft tissue (some fibers of glutei) is interposed between the pelvis and upper end of femur to produce a false movable, painless but unstable hip joint. Postoperatively immobilization is given in extension and neutral rotation for 3—4 weeks, so as to produce fibrous union and some degree of stability. During the immobilization phase, static gluteal, static quadriceps, Ankle foot toe movement should be encouraged. As pain subsides/after stitch removal, active assisted nonweight bearing hip knee movements can be initiated. After 3—4 weeks, nonweight bearing crutch gait can be started. Partial weight bearing in toe-touch position can start after 6 weeks. One should practice isometric gluteal and resisted thera-band abduction exercise and partial weight bearing gait throughout remaining part of life. On weight bearing, the unstable hip joint tends to migrate upward resulting in gradual shortening, which may require foot wear compensation. Some recommend ischial weight relieving orthosis but it is relatively heavier, so people usually discard it due to high energy consumption.

Replacement arthroplasty

- Hemiarthroplasty—In which usually the femoral component (Head and neck) is replaced by the prosthesis.
- **Total hip replacement arthroplasty** —In which both the femoral and acetabular components are replaced. It may be resurfacing, that is, acetabular cavity and head of femur are shaved by excising the articular cartilage and subchondral bone, so as to accommodate the thin acetabular and femoral cup. The acetabular component is usually made up of plastic material and femoral component is metallic and snugly fitted over the respective bony components. **Austin Moore's Prosthesis** is a porous prosthesis whereas **Thompson's Prosthesis** is fixed by bone cement. The metallic femoral component is encased within the plastic acetabular component which can move freely in all directions.

There are 2 techniques

- The prosthesis is fixed by acrylic bone cement which becomes fixed immediately.

- The porous prosthesis is fixed by using screw/nut and bolt. It requires immobilization for about 3 weeks. Healing occurs as ingrowth of the new bones through the pore lock the prosthesis, so it is known as self retaining prosthesis.

There are 2 approaches

- Anterolateral
- Posterior/Posterolateral

Anterolateral—Technically difficult. It requires trochanteric osteotomy to access the hip joint and put the prosthesis. Following replacement GT is fixed by wiring. Postoperatively active hip abduction should be avoided. The prosthesis is stable in flexion (sitting), unstable in extension (standing) therefore immediate postoperatively, patient can be made to sit but standing is deferred by 4–5 days.

Posterior—Technically easy but there is chance of infection. The prosthesis is stable in extension (standing). Patient can be made to stand on second day and sitting should be deferred by 4–5 days.

Indications

- Osteoarthritis
- Fracture neck of femur
- RA
- AVN of head of femur
- Ankylosing spondylitis
- Nonunion neck of femur

Postop complications

- Infection
- DVT
- Loosening of prosthesis

Preop Evaluation—Check the posture, body built, gait, use of walking aid and assistive devices, activities of daily living, hip ROM, muscle power, tightness, contracture, deformity, LLD, movement of spine, pain, cardiovascular, and respiratory evaluation, etc.

Pre-op Physiotherapy—Explain the patient regarding the surgical procedure, expected postop outcome, complication, do's and don'ts, etc. patient must be cautioned against adduction past midline, external-rotation and flexion beyond 90. One should avoid swinging the leg unsupported (pendular exercises), sitting on low height chair, etc.

Preoperative physiotherapy includes deep breathing exercise, effective huffing, coughing, ROM EX, stretching, strengthening and endurance exercises, active ankle foot toe movements, U/L strengthening, static quadriceps, active assisted hip knee flexion-extension, assisted hip abduction, etc.

Teach postop PT protocol—Positioning, turning at regular interval, chest PT, active ankle foot toe movements (DVT prevention), etc.

Postoperative physiotherapy

In case of cemented arthroplasty

Zero day—Patient is in supine lying position with the hip in neutral rotation, slight abduction by placing wedge or pillow between the thighs. Derotational splint may be used to prevent external-rotation of the hip. Deep breathing exercise, effective huffing, and coughing etc. are given to prevent chest complications. Active ankle foot toe movements should be encouraged to prevent circulatory complications like deep vein thrombosis. Turn the patient to quarter turn toward supine, side lying with pillow between the thigh and quarter turn toward prone to prevent accumulation of secretion in the dependent lung segment.

First day—Patient can lie in supine lying position, static quadriceps, and gluteal exercises, assisted hip-knee flexion by sliding the heel on the couch, assisted abduction from abducted position. Abduction is deferred by a few days if the GT is detached and fixed by wiring. Back rest inclination may be gradually increased to about 45°.

Second day—Patient is made to stand through the operated side with the operated limb supported in abduction and neutral rotation. Patient changes to lying perpendicular to long axis of bed by pivoting around the buttock then shifts forward to the edge of the bed. With the buttock resting at the edge of the bed, lower the lower limb while the trunk raises proportionately by U/L support till the foot become flat on the ground and trunk erect. Patient stands with the support of walking frame and made to practice weight transfer and balance. Sideways rocking, forward-backward rocking in standing. Forward–backward rocking in walk standing etc. are practiced so that walking can be initiated by four to five postop days.

Patient can be made to sit in an appropriate height chair. Low height chair result in hyper flexion of hip which is contraindicated. Patient can lie in prone, rolling through the sound side between 7 and 12 days. Regular lying in prone helps in prevention of hip flexion deformity. Walking with a pair of elbow crutches can be initiated between 5 and 7 days and step climbing between 7 and 12 days. While ascending progression to the sound leg with two foot/step and while descending progression with operated limb. Patient is discharged once he learns independent crutch walking, step climbing, sitting, standing etc. while standing, sit with foot flat on the ground with normal BOS, affected operated limb little forward, extend the lumbar spine, bend from the hip joint so that, tip of the great toe, bend knee and eye remain in a straight line, then gets off with hand support.

Review after 6 weeks, when bilateral elbow crutches are replaced by single walking stick. One uses the walking stick on opposite side up to 3 months. After 3 months, flexion beyond 90, adduction past midline can be initiated to put on the shoe, socks, etc. that require hyper flexion, one may use the assistive device and OT interventions.

In case of uncemented arthroplasty

Zero day—Patient is immobilized with hip in slight abduction and neutral rotation for about 4 weeks with the help of derotational splint and wedge in between the thighs. Immediately postoperative encourage patient to do deep breathing exercises, effective huffing - coughing and active ankle foot toe movements.

From **first day** onwards, static quadriceps and from **second/third** day static gluteal exercises can be initiated. Active assisted hip knee flexion extension and abduction can be initiated after stitch removal. Nonweight bearing walking can be initiated after stitch removal. After about **4 weeks**, progressive strengthening exercises and ROM exercises should be given. Partial weight bearing gait can be started after 6 weeks. Walking by single stick starts after 3 months which can be discarded after 4−6 months.

Synovectomy

Joint synovectomy is the surgical removal of the synovial membrane that lines the joint capsule. Synovium surrounds the joints that produce synovial fluid to help lubricate the joint enabling smooth movement. A normal synovium is usually 1 or 2 cell layers thick. In cases of joint disease, the synovium becomes inflamed, proliferated too bulky and produces excess synovial fluid containing an enzyme that can eat away the articular cartilage on the joint surface leading to bone.

A synovectomy is a surgical procedure used to treat synovitis and arthritis that primarily affect the synovium. Synovectomy helps to relieve joint pain and improve the range of motion and ability to function. Inflammatory arthritis with swelling and pain is associated with synovial proliferation [5].

In patients with inflammatory arthritis, excessive growth of synovium is part of an abnormal immune response in which the body recognizes cartilage as a foreign substance that must be attacked. Loss of cartilage eventually leads to damage to the joint surface as well as the stiffness and pain characteristic of all types of arthritis.

Patients who don't respond to medical treatment may be considered for synovectomy before the articular cartilage is involved. The amount of inflamed synovium removed varies from patient to patient, depending on the amount of damage. Some patients require only a particle synovectomy, and others may need a complete synovectomy. Synovectomy may be performed either as an open surgical procedure or with the aid of an *arthroscope*, in which the orthopedic surgeon uses miniaturized instruments, fiberoptic technology and a tiny camera inserted through very small incisions in the skin. Magnified pictures from the camera are projected onto a television monitor in the operating suite, guiding the surgeon throughout the procedure. The surgeon makes a few small incisions around the joint. In one incision, the arthroscope is introduced to view the interior of the joint. The other portals are used for the insertion of surgical instruments to remove the inflamed synovium in the joint. A sterile liquid is infused into the joint to help clear the debris. At the end of the procedure, the arthroscope and instruments are removed and the tiny incisions are covered with a bandage.

In the open technique, an incision is made over the affected joint. The joint capsule is exposed and access is gained through the synovial membrane. The lining is removed by scraping and cutting. Incisions are closed with sutures. A dressing pad is applied over the surgical site.

Advantages of arthroscopic synovectomy over open synovectomy include smaller incisions with less scarring, minimal soft tissue trauma, less postoperative pain, lesser infection rate, faster healing, and recovery.

The choice of technique is often dictated by the affected joint. Using arthroscopy avoids the need for large incisions and allows for a faster rehabilitation. It probably offers a more thorough removal of synovial tissue, as well, but it is considerably more time-consuming than open surgery, and in some joints, more technically difficult to perform.

Synovectomy can yield dramatic improvement in function and pain relief. Patients whose *articular* cartilage is largely intact usually experience the best outcomes. The surgery has low complication rates, although postoperative stiffness is common, and more likely to occur after open surgery than after arthroscopy. The stiffness is treated with physical therapy.

What is the recovery process of a synovectomy?

The recovery process varies, depending on which joint is involved, and the size of the incisions required for the procedure. In the case of larger joints, such as hip and knee synovectomy, postoperative range-of-motion exercises are essential, and patients are started on continuous passive motion (CPM) machines as soon as possible after their procedure.

Physical therapy will usually begin after one or 2 days. Working with an appropriate rehabilitation therapist is important to regain flexibility in the joint. After surgery, the patient must continue to take medication to delay recurrence of synovial inflammation in the treated joint, as well as to protect other joints. In some cases, the medication dose may be reduced after successful synovectomy. "The goal is to slow the whole process of synovial overgrowth down and make the medication more effective. Left untreated, the patient will develop more and more synovitis, which can eventually lead to complete destruction of articular cartilage and the need for joint replacement surgery."

Indications

Joint synovectomy is usually recommended when a painful disabling joint condition does not respond to nonsurgical treatments such as rest, medications (NSAIDs) or corticosteroid injections, and physical therapy. It is usually indicated in rheumatoid arthritis, Juvenile chronic arthritis, systemic lupus erythematosus, traumatic synovitis, infection, postinfectious monoarthritis.

Synovectomy has been, for decades, the procedure of choice for patients with uncontrolled RA.

Synovectomy in hemophilic arthritis has been shown to reduce the incidence of recurrent hemarthrosis and the severity of synovitis [6]. This procedure can be accomplished surgically, arthroscopically, or through intraarticular injection of radioactive colloids or chemical substances. Patients should be considered for synovectomy if, despite aggressive conservative measures, persistent hemarthroses continue with ongoing chronic synovitis.

Joint degenerative disorders such as osteoarthritis are an absolute contraindication for joint synovectomy procedure.

Postoperative care

The postsurgical guidelines to be followed after joint synovectomy include rest, that is, limit the use of the affected joint. Activities such as weight bearing activities in cases of lower limb joints, lifting, carrying, twisting, pushing, or pulling, etc. may be restricted with lifestyle and workplace modifications may be recommended by an occupational therapist.

Zero day—Immediate postoperatively, encourage active ankle foot and toes movements to prevent deep vein thrombosis, static quadriceps exercise.

First day—Patellar mobilization, active hip knee flexion by sliding the heel, partial weight bearing as tolerated by the patient with the help of walker or crutches may be initiated. Walking aids is usually discarded by 48−72 h. Progressive Range of Motion exercises, closed kinetic chain exercises such as leg press, wall supported sit up, lunges, progressive stretching, and endurance exercises are given. Patient discharged after stitch removal with full weight bearing. Balance training starts once full weight bearing is possible.

Risks and Complications—As with all surgery, risks and complications can occur. The possible complications following synovectomy include infection, bleeding, nerve and blood vessel damage, damage to bone surface, and no relief of symptoms. Synovium can grow back and may require repeat surgery.

Hip arthroscopy

Hip arthroscopy is also referred to as keyhole surgery or minimally invasive surgery, is performed through very small incisions to evaluate and treat a variety of hip conditions. Arthroscopy is a surgical procedure in which an arthroscope is inserted into a joint. Arthroscopy is a term that comes from two Greek words, arthro meaning joint, and skopein meaning to examine [7]. Arthroscope is a pencil-sized instrument that has a small lens and lighting system at its one end. Arthroscope magnifies and illuminates the structures inside the body with the light that is transmitted through fiber optics. It is attached to a television camera, and the internal structures are seen on the television monitor.

Indications

- Debridement of loose bodies: Bone chips or torn cartilage debris cause hip pain and decreased range of motion and can be removed with hip arthroscopy.

- Removal of adhesions: Adhesions are areas of built-up scar tissue that can limit movement and cause pain.
- Repair of torn labrum: The labrum lines the outer edge of the "socket" or acetabulum to ensure a good fit. Tears can occur in the labrum causing hip pain.
- Removal of bone spurs: Extrabone growth caused by injury or arthritis that damages the ends of the bones cause pain and limited joint mobility.
- Partial synovectomy: Removal of portions of the inflamed synovium (joint lining) in patients with inflammatory arthritis can help to decrease the patient's pain. However, a complete synovectomy requires an open, larger hip incision.
- Debridement of joint surfaces: Conditions such as arthritis can cause the breakdown of tissue or bone in the joint.
- Repair after Trauma: Repair of fractures or torn ligaments caused by trauma.
- Evaluation and diagnosis: Patients with unexplained pain, swelling, stiffness, and instability in the hip that is unresponsive to conservative treatment may undergo hip arthroscopy for evaluation and diagnosis of their condition.

Procedure

Hip arthroscopy is performed under regional or general anesthesia depending on you and your surgeon's preference. Your surgeon will make two or three small incisions about 1/4 inches in length around the hip joint. Through one of the incisions an arthroscope is inserted. Along with it, a sterile solution is pumped into the joint to expand the joint area and create room for the surgeon to work [8].

The larger image on the television monitor allows the surgeon to visualize the joint directly to determine the extent of damage so that it can be surgically treated. Surgical instruments will be inserted through other tiny incisions to treat the problem. After the surgery, the incisions are closed and covered with a bandage.

Advantages—The advantages of hip arthroscopy over the traditional open hip surgery include smaller incisions, minimal trauma to surrounding ligaments, muscles, and tissues, less pain, faster recovery, lower infection rate, less scarring, earlier mobilization, shorter hospital stay.

Risks and Complications—As with any surgery, there are potential risks and complications involved. Possible risks and complications include infection at the surgical incision site or in the joint space, nerve damage which may cause numbness, tingling, pain, and weakness, excess bleeding into the joint, deep vein thrombosis, embolism, etc.

Recovery—One should take some precautions to promote faster recovery and prevent further complications. These include taking medications as prescribed, use of crutches to prevent or limit bearing weight on the operated hip, physical therapy exercises should be performed to restore normal hip function and improve flexibility and strength. Eating a healthy diet and avoiding smoking will help in faster healing and recovery. Avoid activity which involves lifting heavy things or strenuous exercises for first few weeks after surgery.

Postoperative physiotherapy following hip arthroscopy

The patient should be aware that one's rehabilitative responsibilities such as understanding weight bearing precautions, wound care, and use of assistive devices begins before leaving the outpatient area. Many initial exercises can be performed independently, but the patient should understand the importance of beginning isometric contractions at the hip and ankle plantar flexion and dorsiflexion pumps to facilitate lower extremity circulation.

Phase 1: mobility and initial exercise

During the initial phase of rehabilitation, the goals of the program are to protect the repaired tissue, diminish pain and inflammation, restore pain-free range of motion, prevent muscle inhibition, and normalize gait without crutches. The primary constraint during this phase is that of soft tissue healing and avoiding the negative effects of immobilization [9].

The patient's weight bearing status varies depending on the surgeon's findings and the procedure performed. Unless the surgical procedure addressed a pathology that required extensive healing (i.e., labral repair, femoral osteochondroplasty, and pincer acetabuloplasty, microfracture, etc.), foot-flat weight bearing is typically allowed as tolerated in cases of labral debridement, synovial chondromatosis loose body removal, osteoarthritis debridement, septic arthritis debridement, and trochanteric bursectomy, etc. and crutches are discontinued within the first week. In cases where healing is required, the patient may remain on a limited weight bearing status for up to 8–10 weeks.

Although the discomfort associated with arthroscopy might be surprisingly minimal owing to the combination of capsular penetration with the arthroscopic portals and the traction applied to the capsule during the procedure, there can be significant reflex inhibition. In a typical arthroscopic procedure, the anterolateral and posterolateral portals pass through gluteus medius muscle resulting in limited or poor muscle function-unsupported side pelvic control by the stance side gluteus medius during ambulation. Clinically, it is common for the patient to have a difficult time regaining muscle tone and function postsurgery. Additionally, the short moment arm of the gluteus medius causes a large joint compression force during the single-limb stance phase of gait. In a patient with hip articular pathology, it is common to find inhibition of the gluteus medius because of pain. Consequently, assistive devices are helpful to minimize the Trendelenburg pelvis drop and reestablish a normal gait pattern with synchronous muscle activity.

Early range of motion is initiated to decrease the likelihood of adhesions forming about the joint. Joint motion is normalized by restoring capsular extensibility, with emphasis on passive internal rotation and flexion to prevent scarring between the hip joint capsule and the acetabular labrum. Limitation of hip flexion and internal rotation can occur because of posterior capsular tightness. Stretching of the posterior hip capsule can be achieved through quadruped rocking, that is, prone kneeling to kneel sitting. Exercises are directed in all planes of hip motion, and the end ranges for motion are determined by the patient's level of discomfort. An exception to this rule may be after excision of large bony osteophytes that created a block to motion. Aggressive early stretching under these circumstances can regain the previously blocked motion and might indeed improve function.

Manual mobilization techniques can assist in the reduction of compressive forces across the articular surfaces, lessening discomfort and enhancing cartilage healing [9]. Small accessory oscillatory movements stimulate joint mechanoreceptors that assist in pain modulation while helping to maintain capsular mobility. Graded mobilization with flexion and adduction movement or internal rotation should be gently implemented with the moderately painful joint. Stationary bicycling with minimal to no resistance is an excellent adjunct to the range of motion program and should be done daily. Caution must be taken to not use a recumbent bike or bend over in the aerodynamic riding position to minimize the extreme of hip flexion.

Distraction techniques (longitudinal movement) are most useful when hip movements are painful. Oscillatory longitudinal movements are produced by gently pulling on the lower extremity down the long axis of the femur. This technique can be assisted by a rolling or sliding motion with support under the patient's thigh in the direction of the treatment movement, and it can be performed in varying degrees of hip flexion. In addition, capsular stretching can be specific with three-dimensional mobilization by rotating the femur into the restrictive barrier and performing a longitudinal or inferior glide. Oscillatory movements in a compression mode, stopping short of the painful position, can be helpful, especially for weight bearing pain [10].

Very little anterior-posterior movement takes place within the acetabulum, but anterior and posterior glides can be beneficial for the modulation of pain through the stimulation of joint mechanoreceptors. Glides can also be used as an accessory movement at the limit of physiological range to increase motion of the joint. The presence of a capsular hip pattern is often secondary to a postoperative effusion: a gross limitation of flexion, abduction, and internal rotation with minimal loss of extension and external rotation. Regardless of the pattern of restriction, every attempt should be made to restore full capsular mobility and a physiologic range of motion. In cases with painful restricted motion, the clinician must carefully assess the end feel to motion and the physical status of the joint to determine whether mobilization techniques are a treatment option.

The prevention of muscle inhibition can be achieved through muscle-toning exercises performed within the first week after surgery. Progression depends on the patient's tolerance and should not be overly aggressive. Isometric exercises are the simplest and least likely to aggravate the joint and include sets for the gluteals, quadriceps, hamstrings, adductor, abductor, and lower abdominal muscle groups. Isometric contraction of the antagonistic muscle group may inhibit spasms and promote pain relief. Because of reflex inhibition, emphasis should be placed on isolating and strengthening the gluteal muscles. Assessment of gluteal muscle weakness can best be accomplished with standardized manual muscle-testing procedures in the side-lying and prone positions. The dynamic quality of single-leg support as a part of the kinetic chain can be functionally assessed with a single-leg squat. The single-limb squat test requires frontal plane stability of the pelvis and control of the lower limb in the frontal and transverse planes, both of which require high gluteus medius muscle activation. The single-leg squat test also activates the gluteus maximus muscle. The motion of the single-limb squat requires stability of the lumbo-pelvic region while providing eccentric control of hip flexion and concentric hip extension.

Gluteal isometrics in a neutral pelvic position may decrease spasm of the iliopsoas and provide a decrease in anterior hip pain. The clam shell progression is used to emphasize internal rotation while strengthening the gluteus [11]. It begins with the patient positioned in the side-lying position with the hips flexed approximately 30° feet together, while he or she externally rotates the hip, activating the posterior fibers of the gluteus medius. Progression is achieved by keeping the knees together and performing hip internal rotation (reverse clam shell) activating the anterior and middle portions of the gluteus medius. Further gluteus medius activation is accomplished by abducting and isometrically holding the upper thigh parallel with the floor while performing internal hip rotation. During this phase, patients can start double-leg bridging, limited arc leg press, and mini squats for the gluteus maximus. Previous research has indicated that muscle activation greater than 50%—60% maximum voluntary isometric contraction is considered adequate for muscle strengthening.

An aquatic program is often beneficial for allowing early return to exercise, and it can begin as soon as the portal sites have healed and the sutures have been removed. A pool program allows for muscle relaxation, encouraging joint mobilization and gentle strengthening in a reduced-weight environment. The water buoyancy provides safe resistance, gait progression in waist-deep water, and assistance to movement in all planes. To progress to the intermediate phase, patients should achieve close to full range of motion, a normalized gait pattern without crutches, and minimal to no pain.

Phase 2: intermediate exercise and stabilization

The intermediate phase of rehabilitation typically begins at week 4. Range of motion exercises should be continued until full pain-free range of motion is achieved and while strengthening and stabilization exercises are advanced. Weightbearing and a progressive resistance exercise program such as step up, the band exercises can be added during this phase. Emphasis should be on the elimination of muscle imbalances and motor substitution patterns that occur with activities of daily living. The most common cause for muscle imbalance is chronic overuse or injury, which leads to neuromuscular compromise and an eventual change in the elasticity of the muscle [9]. The neuromuscular compromise can manifest by three mechanisms:

- **Arthrokinetic inhibition**: When a muscle is inhibited by joint dysfunction overuse leads to shortening and tightening (not spasm) of postural muscles, and disuse, to a weakening and inhibition of phasic muscles;

- **Synergistic dominance**: When synergists, stabilizers, and neutralizers overcome a weak or inhibited prime mover; and
- **Reciprocal inhibition**: When a tight muscle decreases neural drive to its functional antagonist, leading to compensation and predictable injury patterns.

The most common muscle imbalance seen clinically is tightness of the hip flexors and erector spinae muscles with weakness of the gluteals and abdominals, resulting in anterior pelvic tilt with increased lumbar lordotic curve. Therefore, core stabilization exercises progress in conjunction with the hip progressive resistive exercise program.

Addressing the proximal stabilizing musculature of trunk and pelvis is an important, often overlooked, aspect of hip rehabilitation; it is critical for optimizing performance and minimizing reinjury risk. Side plank core stabilization exercises with hip abduction results in strengthening emphasize the trunk musculature for improved pelvic stability and abdominal control. Patients often develop the strength, power, and endurance of specific extremity muscles required for activities but are deficient in lumbopelvic-hip complex strength. The core stabilization system should be assessed and challenged as part of the rehabilitation program.

The pelvic tilt test is performed in forward bend position and check for mobility of the hips and lumbar spine; it also controls pelvic posture, which links the upper and lower body. The test begins with tilting the pelvis forward and backward, arching the back (anterior pelvic tilt), and then flattening the lower back (posterior pelvic tilt). The quality and degree of movement indicate the frequency of day-to-day use.

The pelvic rotation test is performed in standing with the foot shoulder width apart and determines the ability of the patient to rotate the lower body independently from the upper. This requires good mobility of the spine, hips, and pelvis, as well as good trunk stability. Check for smooth lateral movement without lateral pelvis motion. This test requires hip rotators and oblique abdominals to rotate the pelvis.

The torso rotation test is performed in standing with the foot shoulder width apart and checks the ability of the patient to rotate the upper body independently from the lower. This movement requires good mobility of the trunk and stability of the hips and pelvis. There should be no motion below the waistline.

The unilateral bridging evaluates stability in the pelvic, lumbar, and core musculature especially, the gluteal. This test highlights gluteus maximus weakness with over recruitment of synergistic muscles such as hamstrings and erector spinae muscles in the lower back. If the unsupported pelvis side drops or the support leg shakes, this indicates gluteal weakness on the support side. If the support leg hamstrings or lower back muscles cramp, this indicates gluteal inhibition. The most common reason for a failed test is gluteal deactivation. The hamstrings and lower back muscles are used for hip extension; they become hyperactive when going into a bridge position and when the leg is extended, a position that is easy for the gluteals to support [12]. If the gluteals are inhibited, cramping will usually occur in the synergistic muscles. Weakness in the abdominals, hamstrings, and gluteals can produce a positive test result.

An integrated functional core stabilization system with a strong lumbopelvic-hip complex will allow for the efficient distribution of weight and absorption and transfer of compressive forces.

Phase 3: advanced exercise and neuromotor control

Proprioceptive deficits routinely occur in conjunction with articular injuries. The acetabular labrum contains free nerve endings and sensory organs, which may contribute to nociceptive and proprioceptive mechanisms. The acetabular labrum improves the stability of the hip joint by maintaining a negative intraarticular pressure. With injury, negative pressure may be lost and stability of the hip compromised by inhibition of normal motor response. Proprioceptive retraining should reestablish neuromotor control, including proprioception and dynamic joint stability. Joint-positioning tasks performed early in the rehabilitative process can enhance proprioceptive and kinesthetic awareness, whereas advanced proprioceptive neuromuscular techniques in functional patterns of movement and modified ranges may be acceptable transitional exercises depending on hip symptoms and status.

Dynamic stabilization exercises encourage muscular cocontractions to balance joint forces [13]. Closed chain methods allow progressive weight bearing transference to the lower extremity that lessens the shear and translational forces across the joint surface. Simple static balance maneuvers in full stance can evolve to single-limb stance, with and without visual input. Progression is then to a combination of balance and strength activities: bilateral heel raises and mini squats to unilateral heel raises and mini squats. More advanced closed kinetic exercises (partial squats, lunges, and dynamic weight shifts) should be initially performed in the pool. Low-force, slow-speed, and controlled activities may transition to high-force, fast-speed activities if the joint allows. Balance devices, mini trampolines, and creative upper extremity activities with balancing can further challenge the neuromuscular system, emphasizing balance and functional training with core stabilization and proper gluteus medius recruitment.

Static, transitional, and dynamic stabilization are phases of progression—from closed chain loading to conscious motion control with high joint tolerance and, ultimately, unconscious control with loading of the joint. Depending on tolerance, the exercise program may progress from slow to fast, simple to complex, stable to unstable, low to high force, and general to specific.

Phase 4: return to activity

The time frame for return to function depends on the hip pathology present and the specific demands of the anticipated activities. Depending on the extent of hip pathology and the surgical procedure, compressive forces generated by physical and sports activities may need to be modified.

Rehabilitation following hip arthroscopy—a systemic review by Jeffry S. Grzybowski, Philip malloy, Catherine stegemnn, Charles Bush—Joseph, Joshua david

Harris and Shane J. Nho, shows rehabilitation protocols were variable in literature [14]. Allowance of immediate weight bearing as tolerated following surgery was reported in seven studies when treatment was labral debridement, synovial chondromatosis loose body removal, osteoarthritis debridement, septic arthritis debridement, and trochanteric bursectomy. When labral repair, femoral osteochondroplasty, and pincer acetabuloplasty were performed, a partial weight-bearing protocol was initiated. Three studies described partial weight bearing as "foot-flat," while two described it as "toe-touch" or "touchdown." Performance of microfracture warranted partial weight bearing for 4—8 weeks in four studies. Use of CPM was reported in only three studies, with between 4 and 12 h/day use for between 4 and 8 weeks. Brace/orthosis use was reported in only four studies: one study denied the use of a brace, two reported only the duration of time used (10 days, 6 weeks), and the other one did report the duration (10—21 days) and motion restrictions (prevent hip extension and external rotation) and situation (while ambulating). Antirotational boot use was reported in only four studies: one study denied their use, and the other three only reported the duration of time used (10 days, 2 and 3 weeks). Only five studies reported the permission and progression to return-to-sport protocols. Initiation of low-impact sports began at 6 weeks at the earliest and high-impact sports between 3 and 6 months. Four studies recommended specific phase-based rehabilitation protocols following hip arthroscopy. All four studies described four phases that generally reported formal timeline-based and criteria-based protocols with precautions advised during each phase [15]. Phase I was a period of protection, between 0 and 6 weeks following surgery, with limited weight bearing, restoration of early motion, limited core abdominopelvic, and hip isometric strengthening, with avoidance of excessive hip extension (beyond neutral), external rotation, deep flexion, and iliopsoas tendonitis. Phase II was a period of advancement to pain-free normal weight bearing and gait and motion, between 4 and 12 weeks postoperatively. Recommendations were for continued strengthening of core and hip muscles, while still avoiding hip flexor tendonitis. Phase III ranged between 8 and 20 weeks after surgery, with focus on endurance, in addition to strength, and progression to sport-specific training. Advancement to Phase IV generally required pain-free full motion, strength, without any subjective or objective deficits during training. Phase IV began at a minimum of 12 weeks following surgery, with progression to safe and unrestricted return to normal activities and sports as well as avoidance of any regression to pain, stiffness, or weakness. All four studies also described a permission to return to running and unrestricted sports protocols. One study reported an explicit requirement of passage of a return-to-sport test to permit running and a different study reported an explicit requirement of passage of a test to permit unrestricted return to sports.

Hip arthrodesis

Arthrodesis is the surgical fusion of joint surfaces, commonly in the knee, spine, or hip. The process may include inserting surgical pins, plates and screws for permanent support. The goal of arthrodesis is to restore, strengthen, and stabilize a weak hip joint. However, replacement arthroplasty is commonly performed and arthrodesis is performed on rare occasions. For many years, arthrodesis was the only option in a severely arthritic or injured hip that limit hip motion resulting undue stress the back or knee muscles and bones. Indications of hip arthrodesis include arthritis, osteoarthritis, osteoporosis, tuberculous arthritis, etc. Patient is too ill for a hip replacement, had a failed hip replacement, hip replacement has become infected, elderly and a hip replacement isn't ideal for your lifestyle, an infection of the femoral head preventing hip replacement, too young with a lifestyle or job where you'd wear out an artificial joint very quickly, history of intravenous substance abuse, which may cause a hip replacement infection. It is a salvage option for a failed THA, and for young active laborers with painful unilateral ankylosis after infection or trauma, neuropathic arthropathy, tumor resection, etc. Spontaneous hip fusions occur following childhood sepsis, ankylosing spondylitis or secondary to heterotopic bone.

Total hip replacement has a good outcome for most patients [16]. However, arthrodesis is an option if you can't tolerate a complex hip replacement.

The arthrodesis surgery fuses the femur to the pelvis with a large plate and screws—eliminating the joint. AO cobra plating is often used, which is stable but disrupts abductors. Transarticular sliding hip screw is inserted across the joint and just superior to the dome of the acetabulum. Disadvantage of this technique includes poor fixation due to large lever arm and the resulting torque on the lever arm and need for postoperative hip spica cast immobilization. The result is a single bone from the pelvis to the knee. A bone graft may be necessary to fill in an area. It takes a long time to heal. Ideal hip fusion position is 20—35° of flexion, 0—5° adduction, 5—10° external rotation and limb-length discrepancy <2 cm are essential for a successful, long-term result. It optimizes the functions and limits effect on adjacent joints. This position minimizes excessive lumbar spine motion and opposite knee motion which helps minimize pain in these regions. Avoid abduction as it creates pelvic obliquity and increased back pain [17]. Lateral approach with trochanteric osteotomy is preferred. It is important to preserve the abductor complex, avoid injury to the superior gluteal nerve. Anterior approach to hip is also popular.

It reduces efficacy of gait by 50%, increases pelvic rotation of contralateral hip, increases stress at adjacent joints, increases oxygen consumption, requires 30% more energy expenditure for ambulation, and average walking speed reduces by 84% of normal gait velocity.

Contraindications includes active infection, severe limb-length discrepancy greater than 2.0 cm, bilateral hip arthritis, adjacent joint degenerative changes in lumbar spine, contralateral hip, ipsilateral knee, severe osteoporosis, contralateral THA, increased failure rate (40%) in THA when there is a contralateral hip arthrodesis. Complications of hip arthrodesis include low back pain, ipsilateral knee degeneration, and contralateral hip degeneration.

Conversion of fusion to THA is indicated in severely debilitating back pain, severe ipsilateral knee pain, with instability, severe contralateral hip pain.

Twenty years after surgery, 80% of patients with hip arthrodesis performed at relatively young age were working and satisfied with their results.

Pre**requisites for hip arthrodesis are** normal contralateral hip, ipsilateral knee, and a **low back, no cardiovascular pathology**.

Osteotomy

Osteotomy is a surgical corrective procedure used to obtain a correct biomechanical alignment of the extremity, so as to achieve equivocal load transmission performed with or without removal of portion of the bone. First femoral osteotomy was performed by John-Rhea, Barton in 1826 when tried to secure the motion of ankylosed hip [18]. In 1835 Sourvier performed first subtrochanteric osteotomy for the treatment of CDH. In 1854 Langen Back introduced subcutaneous osteotomy of femur. In 1918 & 1919 Von Vaeyer and Lorenz described bifurcation operation of upper femoral osteotomy to secure stability in old CDH. In 1922 Sehanz reported low subtrochanteric abduction osteotomy. In 1935 Pauwels described intertrochanteric osteotomy for adduction deformity. In 1936 Mc.Murry performed oblique displacement osteotomy for osteoarthritis of hip and nonunion fracture neck of femur. In 1955 Chiari performed pelvic osteotomy for coverage of the head of the femur in CDH. Blount and Moore described blade plate fixation in high subtrochanteric osteotomy [19].

Osteotomy increases the area of contact and congruity, improves coverage of head of femur, position normal articular cartilage into weight bearing zone, and restores biomechanical advantages.

Based on the location of the osteotomy, it is classified into corrective and compensatory osteotomies. Based on the configuration of the bone cut it is classified into transverse, oblique, crescentic, and displacement osteotomy. Transverse osteotomy is ideal for correction of rotation in myofascial and diaphyseal regions. It is easy to perform. However, it is unstable, not suitable for interfragmentary compression, difficult to control angular correction, requires extensive exposure and periosteal stripping.

Oblique osteotomy provides better bending and rotational stability. It is easily compressed with interfragmentary lag screw. It is especially useful in metaphyseal area. Crescentic osteotomy provides good bony contact and preserves the femoral length. But it is technically difficult. It is useful in varus and valgus deformity. Displacement osteotomy consists of transverse metaphyseal osteotomy, the particular fragment is rotated and impacting one corner of the metaphysis into medullary canal of the other fragment. It changes bending and loading force into compressive load, preserving bone length and joint alignment.

Contraindication of osteotomy includes neuropathy, arthropathy, inflammatory arthropathy, active infection, advanced arthritis, ankylosis, osteoporosis, advanced age, obesity, and smoking, etc.

Osteotomy around the hip joint involved proximal femoral osteotomy, pelvic osteotomy. Proximal femoral osteotomy is classified according to displacement of distal fragment, anatomical location of osteotomy, and indication.

Displacement of distal fragment are two types—Transpositional and angulation osteotomy.

In transpositional osteotomy longitudinal axis of distal fragment remains parallel to the longitudinal terminal axis of proximal fragment [19]. It is used in fracture neck of femur and osteoarthritis, for example, Mc.murry's osteotomy, Pauwel's osteotomy, and Putti's osteotomy. In angulation osteotomy longitudinal axis of distal fragments forms an angle with that of proximal fragment. It is used in fixed flexion deformity, abduction/adduction osteotomy.

Depending on the anatomical site femoral osteotomy is divided into high-cervical, intertrochanteric, greater-trochanteric, and subtrochanteric osteotomy.

Based on the indication the osteotomies are classified as follows:

1. Fracture nonunion neck of femur: McMurry's osteotomy, Dickson osteotomy, Putti's osteotomy, Schanz osteotomy.
2. Osteoarthritis: Pauwel's valgus/varus osteotomy, Mc.Murry osteotomy.
3. Unstable intertrochanteric fracture: Dimon-Hughston osteotomy, Sarminento's osteotomy.
4. Unreduced CDH: Lorenz bifurcation osteotomy, Schanz osteotomy, Low sub-trochanteric osteotomy, Penburten acetabuloplasty.
5. Congenital coxavalga—vara: Cuneiform osteotomy by Fish, Pauwel's Y osteotomy, Valgus osteotomy, Basilar osteotomy.
6. Leg calve Perthe's disease: Varus derotation osteotomy, Salter osteotomy, Chairi osteotomy.
7. AVN of the head of the femur: Sugioka trans-trochanteric osteotomy, Varus derotation osteotomy.
8. Slipped capital femoral epiphyses: Close wedge osteotomy of neck of femur includes technique of Fish, technique of Dunn just distal to slip, base of neck technique by Kramer et al., technique of Abraham et al. [20] Compensatory osteotomy include ball and socket osteotomy, biplanner osteotomy.
9. Osteotomies in paralytic hip disorder: Varus osteotomy, Rotation osteotomy, Extension osteotomy.

Osteotomies of pelvis are divided into:

 (i) Single innominate (salter osteotomy),
 (ii) Double innominate (Sutherland),
 (iii) Triple innominate (Steel osteotomy), Peri acetabular (Wagner osteotomy), Ganz osteotomy.

Postop physiotherapy

Casting: Double hip spica cast for 6 weeks, nonweight bearing.

Healing Time: Approximately 6—8 weeks.

Precautions: Avoid aggressive/forceful range of motion initially -Children who were nonweight bearing preop may be osteopenic and fixation of the surgical hardware may be limited. Special care must be taken during exercise and progressive weight bearing activities contraindications: No impact, torque or unprotected weight bearing for the first 6 weeks postop—minimize risk for falling.

Phase 1: post-op day 1—7

Goals: Protect surgical site, both skin incision and bony healing—Non weight bearing—Address splinting, bracing, and equipment needs—Address and instruct patient and family in safe mobility and transfers for daily function and hygiene.

Pain management which may include use of ice, heat, massage and/or electrical stimulation for pain modulation only.

PROM, AAROM of the knees and ankles -isometric contraction of the gluts, quads and hamstrings -Patient and family are able to demonstrate understanding of post-op precautions and home exercise program.

Criteria to Progress: Safe mobility and transfers for completion of ADLs.

Phase 2: post-op day 8—21

Goals: Pain management as needed.

Criteria to Progress: Ongoing healing of surgical sites, independent with transfers, ADLs and mobility.

Phase 3: post-op day 22 to end of 6 weeks

Goals: Avoid impact, torque and reduce risk for falling, re-evaluate splinting and bracing needs for assistance with gait efficiency at the end of postop week six if weight bearing is allowed by the surgeon.

Criteria to Progress: Ongoing healing of surgical site.

Heterotopic bone (HO)

Heterotopic bone formation is the extraarticular bone formation that occurs in skeletal muscles, subcutaneous tissues, fibrous tissues, and usually does not involve the periosteum [21].

HO was first described by Patin in 1692 while working with children diagnosed with myositis ossificans progressiva. In 1918, Dejerine & Ceillier detailed the anatomical, clinical, and histological features of ectopic bone formation in soldiers who sustained spinal injuries during World War I [22]. Marshall Urist described the osteoinducive properties of bone morphogenic protein in ectopic areas such as muscle, which is still considered a "landmark discovery" in orthopedic research [23].

Causes: the exact cause is not known. The primitive mesenchymal cells in connective tissue transformation into osteoblastic tissue are usually predisposed by trauma and surgery. Following traumatic brain injury, systemic factors such as bone morphogenetic factors, growth hormone, basic fibroblast growth factor, etc. are released, whereas in case of fracture local stimulating factors are released that stimulate mesenchymal stem cells to differentiate and osteoblast formation. HO also develops in cases of deep burn.

Although HO can be found at any site, it is most prevalent in the major joints such as the hip, elbow, shoulder, and knee.

Posttraumatic HO begins with spindle cell proliferation within the first week of the traumatic event. Within 1−2 weeks, primitive osteoid develops. After the second week, primitive cartilage and woven bone can be seen. Trabecular bone forms 2−5 weeks after the trauma. Amorphous calcium phosphate is gradually replaced by hydroxyapatite crystals as the mineralization progresses. After about 6 months, there is an appearance of true bone in the connective tissue between the muscle planes. Posttraumatic HO commonly involves the brachialis muscle following fracture, dislocation of elbow.

Neurogenic heterotopic ossification occurs after sickle cell anemia, hemophilia, tetanus, poliomyelitis, multiple sclerosis, and toxic epidermal necrolysis. Neurogenic HO develops only in sites distal to the level of the spinal cord injury often develop in hip and quadriceps muscles. The areas affected by HO are almost always on the affected side of brain injury or stroke.

Postsurgical HO most commonly develops after procedures which require open reduction, internal fixation, and joint replacement surgeries, with THA being the most common. HO may also occur following lower extremity amputation.

Genetic forms include two types: Fibrodysplasia Ossificans Progressiva and Progressive Osseous Heteroplasia. These types are described as massive deposits of heterotopic bone around multiple joints in the absence of an inciting event (i.e., trauma). This is the most severe type of HO, progressively forming throughout the life and severely affecting health, life expectancy, and quality of life [24].

Reactive lesions of the hands and feet are usually associated with the periosteum or periarticular fibrous tissue, which differentiates the category from myositis ossificans.

The most common conditions found in conjunction with heterotopic ossification includes ankylosing spondylitis, rheumatoid arthritis, hypertrophic osteoarthritis, diffuse idiopathic skeletal hyperostosis, Paget's disease, Quadriplegia, and paraplegia.

Muscle injury due to trauma, forced passive movements for elbow extension in case of fracture, dislocation, forced passive movements to lower extremities and vigorous massage spinal cord injury, brain injury, etc. damage the muscle tissues. The periosteum may be stripped and osteoblasts released. There occurs bleeding following injury that clots and hematoma is formed within the interstitial tissues that may get ossified over time. Initially one complains of pain, swelling, and limitation of movements. Pain may be continuous in nature, aggravates with movements. On palpation warmth, tenderness felt.

Clinical signs and symptoms of HO may appear as soon as 3 weeks or up to 12 weeks after initial musculoskeletal trauma, spinal cord injury, or other precipitating events [25].

Chronology of development of heterotopic ossification

- 0 days: ± erythema, swelling, tenderness
- 7 days: clinically palpable mass
- 7−14 days: poorly defined shadow on radiograph
- 14−21 days: osteoid deposition, radiographic shadows
- 21−35 days: fluffy radiodensities; the "dotted veil" effect
- 24 days: definite radiographic evidence
- 30 days: mineralization shows a zonal pattern (best seen on CT scan)
- 45 days: histologic "zonal" pattern evident, reflecting well-formed mineralization at the periphery
- 180−365 days: development of mature bone

Diagnosis

X-rays cannot detect the mineralization of HO during first weeks after onset. HO seen on radiographs 4−6 weeks postinjury has a typical appearance of circumferential ossification with a lucent center.

Ultrasonography detects HO 2 weeks earlier than by X-ray, which is more accurate than any laboratory tests.

CT may detect soft tissue ossification at earlier stages than standard radiograph.

Three-phase technetium-99m (99mTc) methylene diphosphonate bone scan is most sensitive imaging modality for early detection and assessing the maturity of HO. Can use to monitor the metabolic activity of HO and determine appropriate time for surgery and predict postoperative recurrence. Usually, positive >2 weeks before radiographic evidence of HO.

Prostaglandin E2 (PGE2) is felt to be reliable bone marker for early detection and determining treatment efficacy, monitor PGE2 excretion in 24-h urinalysis.

Alkaline Phosphatase (ALP) is frequently used in early detection of HO. ALP values are increased in early HO and plateau at ∼4 weeks. Cannot be used to draw clinical conclusions about maturity or recurrence of HO.

Brooker classification of heterotopic ossification (following THA) [26]

- Class 1: Island of bone within a soft tissue about the hip.
- Class 2: Bone spurs originating from the pelvis of proximal end of femur leaving at least 1 cm between opposing bone surfaces.
- Class 3: Bone spurs originating from pelvis or proximal femur leaving <1 cm between opposing bone surfaces.
- Class 4: Ankyloses of the hip.

Brooker did not describe a class 0 but subsequent studies using the Brooker classification have defined Class 0 as the absence of radiographic HO.

Schmidt and hackenbrock classification of heterotopic ossification (following THA) [27]

- Region 1: Heterotopic ossification strictly below the tip of the greater trochanter. Region 2: Heterotopic ossification below and above the tip of the greater trochanter. Region 3: Heterotopic ossification strictly above the tip of the greater trochanter.
- Grade A: Single or multiple heterotopic ossification <10 mm in maximal extent without contact with pelvis or femur.
- Grade B: Heterotopic ossification >10 mm without contact with the pelvis but with possible contact with the femur; no bridging from the femur to the proximal part of the greater trochanter; no evidence of ankylosis.
- Grade C: Ankylosis by means of firm bridging from femur to pelvis.

McAfee's classification of heterotopic ossification (following total disc arthroplasty) [28]

- 0: No HO.
- 1: Islands of bone not within the margins of the disc and not interfering with motion.
- 2: Bone within the margins of the disc but not blocking motion.
- 3: Bone within the margins of the disc and interfering with motion of the prosthesis.
- 4: Bone ankylosis.

Management

The treatment of heterotopic ossification is largely dependent on the amount of ectopic bone formation, the location and the associated functional limitations of the patient.

The first goal of medical management is to identify those patients at risk for developing HO and treating them prophylactically. Research supports two other approaches for the medical management of HO: (1) surgical excision and (2) radiation therapy.

Prophylactic Treatment: Further research needs to be done in this area; however, there are currently experimental options. These include

Local radiation therapy: Decreased incidence of all Brooker classes of HO following THA, but has greater effect on preventing Brooker classification three and four compared to NSAIDS.

Physiotherapy

Aim of physiotherapy is to prevent further damage, promote reabsorption of edema, and relieve pain. Initially rest is given with ice, compression, elevation. As rest pain and warmth subsides active pain free movements can be initiated. Heat therapy, ultrasound, massage, passive stretching, or loading the muscle should be avoided.

Sharp's protocol of iontophoresis, ultrasound, and passive movement: Acetic acid iontophoresis is useful before completion of ossification. Myositis consists of calcium carbonate ($CaCO_3$), which is not soluble in normal blood pH level. Acetate binds with calcium forms calcium acetate, which is soluble in blood and removed. 3 mL of 2% acetic acid is placed under the cathode while using direct current, so that acetate ions are repelled into the body tissues that bind with calcium ions and removed. Iontophoresis is followed by pulsed ultrasound that may disperse the acetic acid throughout the myositis site. Then gentle passive movements within pain free range are given. This protocol is administered on alternate days for 3 weeks [29].

Extracorporeal shock wave therapy is a noninvasive low-risk treatment for heterotopic ossification and can be a complement to usual medical treatment, physiotherapy, and before surgery [30].

Medications: Medications are prescribed to patients who are at risk for developing heterotopic ossification for preventive measures and to aid in the treatment after formation of heterotopic lesions.

Nonsteroidal antiinflammatory drugs (NSAIDS): Indomethacin acts directly as inhibition of the differentiation of mesenchymal cells into osteogenic cells and indirectly inhibition of posttraumatic bone remodeling by suppression of prostaglandin-mediated response and antiinflammatory properties.

Biphosphonates: Threefold action includes inhibition of calcium phosphate precipitation, slowing of hydroxyapatite crystal aggregation and inhibition of the transformation of calcium phosphate to hydroxyapatite.

Surgical intervention: The goal of surgical intervention is to align the joint position and to improve joint mobility.

Garland has recommended following criteria for surgical intervention:

- 6 months following traumatic development of HO.
- 1-year following development of HO secondary to a spinal cord injury.
- 18 months following development of HO secondary to head injury.

The above timetables were established to determine the most optimal timing of surgical intervention. Clinicians must determine if the lesion has reached maturation before surgical excision to decrease the risk of intraoperative complications such as hemorrhage, and the reoccurrence of the ectopic lesion. The use of bone scans to determine metabolic activity of the lesion and serum ALP levels are common aids in this decision-making process.

Shehab et al. describe criteria for recommending surgical removal of heterotopic ossification as follows [31]

1. Significantly limited ROM of involved joint (e.g., hip should have <50 deg ROM) for most patients, progression to joint ankylosis is the most serious complication of heterotopic ossification.
2. Absence of local fever, swelling, erythema, or other clinical findings of acute heterotopic ossification.

3. Normal serum alkaline phosphate levels.
4. Return of bone scan findings to normal or near normal; if serial quantitative bone scans are obtained, there should be a sharply decreasing trend followed by a steady state for 2—3 months.

Postoperative rehabilitation

It is recommended that a rehabilitation program should start within the first 24 h after surgery. The program should last for 3 weeks to prevent adhesion. Preoperative physiotherapy includes active free, active assisted, passive range of exercises, and strengthening of muscles around the joint. Isometric muscle contractions around the muscles should be encouraged to prevent muscle atrophy.

Postoperative rehabilitation has also shown to benefit patients with recent surgical resection of heterotopic ossification. The postop management of HO is similar to preop treatment but much more emphasis is placed on edema control, scar management, and infection prevention. Calandruccio et al. outlined a rehabilitation protocol for patients who underwent surgical excision of heterotopic ossification of the elbow [32]. The phases of rehab and goals for each phase are as follows:

Phase I (week 1)

1. Prevent infection
2. Protect and decrease stress on surgical site
3. Decrease pain
4. Control and decrease edema
5. ROM to 80% of affected joint
6. Maintain ROM of joint proximal and distal to surgical site

Phase II (2—8 weeks)

1. Reduce pain
2. Manage edema
3. Encourage limited ADL performances
4. Promote scar mobility and proper remodeling
5. Promote full ROM of affected joint
6. Encourage quality muscle contractions

Phase III (9—24 weeks)

1. Self manage pain
2. Prevent flare-up with functional activities
3. Improve strength
4. Improve ROM (if still limited)
5. Return to previous levels of activity

References

[1] Evans JT, Evans JP, Walker RW, Blom AW, Whitehouse MR, Sayers A. How long does a hip replacement last? A systematic review and meta-analysis of case series and national registry reports with more than 15 years of follow-up. Lancet 2019;393:647−54.

[2] Marshall DA, Pykerman K, Werle J, Lorenzetti D, Wasylak T, Noseworthy T, Dick DA, O'Connor G, Sundaram A, Heintzbergen S, Frank C. Hip resurfacing versus total hip arthroplasty: a systematic review comparing standardized outcomes. Clin Orthop Relat Res 2014;472(7):2217−30.

[3] Liu XW, Zi Y, Xiang LB, Wang Y. Total hip arthroplasty: a review of advances, advantages and limitations. Int J Clin Exp Med 2015;8(1):27−36.

[4] Nilsdotter A, Roos EM, Westerlund JP, Roos HP, Lohmander S. Comparative responsiveness of measures of pain and function after total hip replacement. Arthritis Care Res 2001;45(3):258−62.

[5] Haywood L, McWilliams DF, Pearson CI, Gill SE, Ganesan A, Wilson D, Walsh DA. Inflammation and angiogenesis in osteoarthritis. Arthritis Rheumatol 2003;48(8):2173−7.

[6] Rodríguez-Merchán EC, Goddard N, Lee CA. Chronic haemophilic synovitis. Musculoskeletal aspects of haemophilia. 2nd ed. Madrid, Spain: John Wiley & Sons; 2008. p. 43−9.

[7] Bhattacharyya M, Bradley H. Intraoperative handling and wound healing of arthroscopic portal wounds: a clinical study comparing nylon suture with wound closure strips. J Perioperat Pract 2008;18(5):194−8.

[8] Hsiao MS, Kusnezov N, Sieg RN, Owens BD, Herzog JP. Use of an irrigation pump system in arthroscopic procedures. Orthopedics 2016;39(3):e474−8.

[9] Voight ML, Robinson K, Gill L, Griffin K. Postoperative rehabilitation guidelines for hip arthroscopy in an active population. Sport Health 2010;2(3):222−30.

[10] Griffin KM. Rehabilitation of the hip. Clin Sports Med 2001;20(4):837−50.

[11] Coplen EM, Voight ML. Rehabilitation of the hip. In: Byrd J, editor. Operative hip arthroscopy. New York, NY: Springer; 2013.

[12] Macadam P, Feser EH. Examination of gluteus maximus electromyographic excitation associated with dynamic hip extension during body weight exercise: a systematic review. Int J Sports Phys Ther 2019;14(1):14−31.

[13] HuxelBliven KC, Anderson BE. Core stability training for injury prevention. Sport Health 2013;5(6):514−22.

[14] Grzybowski JS, Malloy P, Stegemann C, Bush-Joseph C, Harris JD, Nho SJ. Rehabilitation following hip arthroscopy − a systematic review. Front Surg 2015;2:21.

[15] Kuhns BD, Weber AE, Batko B, Nho SJ, Stegemann C. A four-phase physical therapy regimen for returning athletes to sport following hip arthroscopy for femoroacetabular impingement with routine capsular closure. Int J Sports Phys Ther 2017;12(4):683−96.

[16] Arden NK, Kiran A, Judge A, Biant LC, Javaid MK, Murray DW, Carr AJ, Cooper C, Field RE. What is a good patient reported outcome after total hip replacement? Osteoarthr Cartilage 2011;19(2):155−62.

[17] Morimoto T, Sonohata M, Kitajima M, Yoshihara T, Hirata H, Mawatari M. Hip-spine syndrome: the coronal alignment of the lumbar spine and pelvis in patients with ankylosed hips. Spine Surg Relat Res 2019;4(1):37−42.

[18] Hernigou P. Earliest times before hip arthroplasty: from john rhea barton to themistocles Glück. Int Orthop 2013;37(11):2313−8.

[19] Varshney MK. Osteotomies around the hip joint. In: Essential orthopedics: principles & practice. 1st ed. New Delhi, India: Jaypee Publishers; 2016.

[20] Mahran MA, Baraka MM, Hefny HM. Slipped capital femoral epiphysis: a review of management in the hip impingement era. SICOT J 2017;3:35.

[21] Meyers C, Lisiecki J, Miller S, Levin A, Fayad L, Ding C, Sono T, McCarthy E, Levi B, James AW. Heterotopic ossification: a comprehensive review. JBMR Plus 2019;3(4): e10172.

[22] Peters N, Baltin CT, Barham M, Wevers A. An unusual finding: heterotopic ossification located in the subcutis of the iliac region — a case report in the context of current literature. Transl. Res. Anat. 2021;25:100137.

[23] Grgurevic L, Pecina M, Vukicevic S. Marshall R. Urist and the discovery of bone morphogenetic proteins. Int Orthop 2017;41(5):1065—9.

[24] Shore EM. Fibrodysplasia ossificans progressiva: a human genetic disorder of extraskeletal bone formation, or—how does one tissue become another? Wiley Interdiscip Rev Dev Biol 2012;1(1):153—65.

[25] Sun E, Hanyu-Deutmeyer AA. Heterotopic ossification. In: StatPearls treasure Island (FL). Seattle, WA: StatPearls Publishing; 2022.

[26] Hug KT, Alton TB, Gee AO. Classifications in brief: Brooker classification of heterotopic ossification after total hip arthroplasty. Clin Orthop Relat Res 2015;473(6): 2154—7.

[27] Schmidt J, Hackenbroch MH. A new classification for heterotopic ossifications in total hip arthroplasty considering the surgical approach. Arch Orthop Trauma Surg 1996; 115:339—43.

[28] McAfee PC, Cunningham BW, Devine J, Williams E, Yu-Yahiro J. Classification of heterotopic ossification (HO) in artificial disk replacement. J Spinal Disord Tech 2003; 16(4):384—9.

[29] Wieder DL. Treatment of traumatic myositis ossificans with acetic acid iontophoresis. Phys Ther 1992;72:133—7.

[30] Reznik JE, Gordon SJ, Barker RN, Keren O, Arama Y, Galea MP. Extracorporeal Shock Wave therapy (ESWT) as a treatment for recurrent neurogenic heterotopic ossification (NHO). Brain Inj 2013;27(2):242—7.

[31] Shehab D, Elgazzar AH, Collier BD. Heterotopic ossification. J Nucl Med 2002;43(3): 346—53.

[32] Hsu JE, Keenan MA. Current review of heterotopic ossification. UPO J 2010;20: 126—30.

Miscellaneous conditions

Congenital dislocation of hip

Another name for Congenital Dislocation of Hip (CDH) is "developmental dysplasia of the hip (DDH)." Although DDH is most often present at birth, it may also develop during a child's first year of life.

The degree of hip looseness, or instability, varies among children with DDH.

- Dislocated: In the most severe cases of DDH, the head of the femur is completely out of the socket.
- Dislocatable: In these cases, the head of the femur lies within the acetabulum, but can easily be pushed out of the socket during a physical examination.
- Subluxatable: In mild cases of DDH, the head of the femur is simply loose in the socket. During a physical examination, the bone can be moved within the socket, but it will not dislocate.

Causes

Exact cause is not known. It is thought to be genetic and familial as ligamentous laxity is genetically *inherited*. Hip dysplasia is often associated with CDH, that is, increased neck shaft angle, shallow acetabulum, increased femoral anteversion which makes the hip joint unstable predisposing to CDH.

- Environmental factors include secretion of relaxin hormone just before delivery, which may cross the placental barrier enhancing the joint laxity and predisposing to CDH. Intrauterine malpositioning, especially breech presentation, Oligohydramnios (low levels of amniotic fluid) is often associated with CDH [1].
- The incidence is more common in female with 3:1 ratio (female 70%, male 30%). Firstborn children are more prone [2]. Left side is more involved than right (left 60%, right 20%) and bilateral 20%.

Pathomechanics

Shallow acetabulum with increased neck shaft angle and anteversion may lead to hip dislocation. The dislocated head displaces upward by the pull of glutei. The head of the femur gets stuck against the pelvic bone resulting in development of false acetabulum on weight bearing.

Secondary soft tissue changes such as shortening of hip flexors, adductors, and joint capsule develop over time which may prevent close reduction. Acetabular labrum gets inverted and deformed resulting in limbus formation [3]. Overtime the joint capsule becomes hour glass in shape. The ligamentum teres often becomes unduly thick and adaptive shortening of hip flexors develop.

Lack of weight bearing results in persistent increase in neck shaft angle, anteversion, and shallow acetabulum. Lack of contact between articular surfaces, alternate compression, and relaxation results in degeneration of articular cartilage.

Clinical feature

All the newborn must be screened to rule out congenital anomalies like CDH, Erb's palsy, AGMC, Torticollis, CTEV, etc. Unilateral CDH is characterized by shortening, high riding GT, asymmetrical skin creases in the inner aspect of thigh, asymmetrical gluteal fold, etc. Emptiness is felt in femoral triangle. Special test like **Ortolani and Barlow**, **Bryant's Triangle, Nelaton's Line, Schoemaker's Line,** etc. are diagnostic of CDH. In bilateral CDH there is widening of perineum, **Bryant's Triangle, Nelaton's Line, Schoemaker's Line,** etc. are diagnostic [4]. In an older child, hip abduction range may be limited. Child may walk in limping and Trendelenburg sign may be positive. X-ray is diagnostic after 4 months of age. X-ray of the hips with the pelvis in A-P view is taken.

- **Shenton's line**—is drawn along the medial neck of femur and inferior margin of superior pubic ramus. Normally both the lines join together to form a smooth curve. In case of CDH this curve is broken [5].
- **Perkin's line**—the H line is a horizontal line drawn through the tri-radiate cartilage of acetabulum, vertical lines are drawn on the outer edges of acetabulum on both the sides. Normally upper femoral epiphysis lies in the lower inner quadrant. In case of CDH, it lies in the upper outer quadrant.
- **Acetabular index**—is the inclination of the roof, that is, the angle formed by the H-line and the inclined line along the roof of acetabulum is about 22° normally. If it is more than 40° suggests shallow acetabulum and CDH [6].
- Secondary changes like false acetabulum may be present in the late stage.

Management

New born within 6 months of age—Retain the hip in abduction and flexion so that the head of the femur will be retained within the acetabulum and becomes stable because of regression of the laxed capsule-ligamentous structure [7]. So, to achieve it various splints are available.

1. Von rosen splint: It is a plastic frame that passes over the shoulder and under the thighs. Both frames are interconnected on the back.

2. Pavlik harness splint: Pavlik harness is most commonly used. It has a chest strap with shoulder harness. This harness presses their hip joints into the sockets. The harness abducts the hip by securing their legs in a froglike position. Anterior and posterior straps extend from the chest strap to hold the foot securely. It allows the child to move the legs freely. So, disuse atrophy and joint stiffness can be avoided. Your baby may wear the harness for 6−12 weeks, depending on their age and the severity of the condition. Your baby may need to wear the harness full time or part time.
3. Craig-nappy splint: it is like a napkin. Adduction prevented.
4. Ilfeld splint: It has thigh bands connected by a cross bar. Adduction prevented, static splint.
5. Broom stick splint: It is a cylindrical long leg plaster cast with a cross bar which held the thighs in abduction and medial rotation.

After 6 months—Adaptive shortening of the soft tissue may prevent close reduction therefore Bryant's/Gallow's traction is used. It is an overhead skin traction that tends to stretch the periarticular soft tissue structure so that gradually hip abduction ROM is increased to obtain the reduction at some point. If it doesn't get reduced by traction itself, close manipulative reduction following traction can be tried up to 18 months of age. After 18 months contracture of joint capsule, hip flexors and adductors and inverted acetabular labrum will prevent close reduction, so open reduction followed by hip spica immobilization for 3 weeks is given.

Close reduction

Maneuvering the hip into the socket, which is called a closed reduction, is done with general anesthesia. Prognosis is less satisfactory, as there is risk of damage to blood vessels supplying head of femur and AVN. To minimize the risk of AVN overhead traction to both the legs with gradual increase in abduction range for 3 weeks is given [8]. If traction doesn't widely abduct the thighs adductor tenotomy may be required followed by reduction under anesthesia can be tried. If reduction feels unstable and X-ray shows unsatisfactory reduction suggest an infolded limbus and require open reduction. Following closed manipulative reduction, hip spica immobilization for 3−6 weeks is given. After 6 weeks the plaster is replaced by Pavlik splint/Denis Brown splint.

Open reduction

In case closed manipulative reduction is not possible then surgery to deal with the inverted limbus followed by reduction is formed. The surgeon will lengthen baby's tendons and remove other obstacles before positioning the hip. This is called an open reduction. After your baby's hip is placed into position, their hips and legs will be in casts for at least 6 weeks.

If your child is 18 months or older or hasn't responded well to treatment, they may need femoral or pelvic osteotomies to reconstruct their hip. This means that a surgeon will divide or reshape the head of their femur (the ball of the hip joint), or the acetabulum of their pelvis (the hip socket).

If diagnosed early and treated successfully, children are able to develop a normal hip joint and should have no limitation in function.

Untreated case above the age limit—Left untreated, DDH can lead to pain and osteoarthritis (OA) by early adulthood. It may produce a difference in leg length or decreased agility. It is unwise to try to reduce the dislocation. The force needed for reduction may damage the hip and a painful stiff hip may develop. If the untreated hip is mobile, there is no pain and patient walks with limping and it should be left like that. The possible techniques above the age limit include innominate osteotomy of Salter, pelvic osteotomy of Chiari, acetabuloplasty, and femoral osteotomy. Salter's innominate osteotomy involves cut and divide above acetabulum, rotate it to cover head of femur and fix the gap with bone grafts.

Chiari's pelvic displacement osteotomy involve cut above acetabulum and displace medially to cover head of femur. In acetabuloplasty cut above the roof of acetabulum and mold it to increase the concavity of the acetabulum. Gap above roof is filled by graft [9].

To correct coxavalga and anteversion, intercondylar medial closed wedge osteotomy to correct coxavalga and derotation to correct anteversion along with internal fixation is done. Following surgery part is immobilized for about 6 weeks. During immobilization active ankle-foot-toe movement, static gluteals and quadriceps must be encouraged. After plaster removal nonweight bearing exercise, preferably hydrotherapy is used to restore the joint mobility and strength before wearing the joint.

Complications

Children treated with spica casting may have a delay in walking. However, when the cast is removed, walking development proceeds normally.

The Pavlik harness and other positioning devices may cause skin irritation around the straps, and a difference in leg length may remain. Growth disturbances of the upper thighbone are rare, but may occur due to a disturbance in the blood supply to the growth area in the thighbone.

Even after proper treatment, a shallow hip socket may still persist, and surgery may be necessary in early childhood to restore the normal anatomy of the hip joint.

Outcomes

Even with appropriate treatment, hip deformity and OA may develop later in life. This is especially true when treatment begins after the age of 2 years.

Slipped capital femoral epiphysis

The upper femoral epiphysis is displaced from its normal position often the femoral neck before it fuses in adolescent years, that is, 12–15 in male, 10–13 in female. The incidence is more common in male with 2:1 ratio. Left side more involved than right. In 20% case, it may be bilateral.

Cause

The exact cause is not known. But it is thought to be associated with familial and genetic involvement. Endocrine dysfunction such as genetic adipose syndrome predisposes to slipped capital femoral epiphysis [10]. Obesity is one of the precipitating factors. Trauma may be one of the causes. In case of trauma the slippage is sudden. In about 70% of cases the slip occurs gradually.

Pathomechanics

Weakness of cartilage junction during adolescence may result in CDH. The growth plate changes from horizontal to an oblique position in adolescence as the neck shaft angle decreases over time. Periosteum of the femur which is the main stabilizer of epiphysis is atrophied at same time. Sudden increase in body weight in adolescent exerts downward pressure over head of femur and upward pull of hip abductor on femur tends to displace the capital femoral epiphysis downward. The epiphysis is displaced downward to neck of femur. If it is left untreated the epiphysis fuses to the neck in an abnormal position giving rise to coxavara. The tension on the circumflex femoral artery may compromise the circulation resulting in AVN and OA.

The growth hormone helps in proliferation of cells of the growth plate and sex hormone helps in end plate closure as skeletal maturity. In case of adipose genital syndrome, deficiency in both hormones weaken the end plate precipitating the slippage [10].

Clinical features

Usually complains of gradual onset of limping. Sudden onset of limping may be associated with history of fall. Child may be overweight, history of familial involvement may be present. Pain refers on front of thigh, the knee, limitation of abduction and internal rotation range present. During flexion, the thigh rolls into abduction and external rotation. Shortening is present. Wasting of glutei, GT may be higher and more posterior than the unaffected side.

X-ray

- **AP view**—shows even trivial changes. The growth plate appears wider. A line drawn along superior surface of the neck remains superior to the head instead of passing through it —**Trethowan's Sign.**
- **Lateral view**—deformity obvious from beginning.

Depending on the extent the slippage is classified into **three types.**

- **Grade 1**—slippage is less than 1/3rd the width of the femoral neck
- **Grade 2**—slippage is in between 1/3rd to 1/2nd the width of the femoral neck
- **Grade 3**—slippage more than 1/2 the width of the femoral neck

In chronic cases sign of new bone formation in the postero-inferior aspect of metaphysis adjacent to femoral head may be seen.

Management

Aim of management includes

- Prevent further slippage by prevent by avoiding weight bearing.
- Reduction of displacement by progressive abduction and internal rotation.
- Stabilization till skeletal maturity takes place.

In case of mild slippage (grade 1), reduction is not attempted. Under image intensifier control epiphysis is fixed using multiple threaded pins. If the operation is delayed give rest by traction. If the displacement is moderate-severe apply traction, slowly and progressively abduct and internally rotate the hip to achieve reduction, then fixation under image intensifier is given. Alternately reduction is achieved by general anesthesia but there is chance of injury to circumflex femoral artery and AVN. Following reduction rest is given for the synovitis, pain, spasm to subside. Then fixation by closed method using threaded pin, free flanged nail, slender screw along the neck of the epiphysis. Open reduction also complicates the AVN; therefore, the epiphysis is fixed in its displaced position using three pins. After a few months of rest, corrective osteotomy is done bringing the head into acetabulum. Usually, lateral wedge osteotomy with derotation and internal rotation is done following surgery immobilization by hip spica in abducted position is given.

Complications

1. **Coxavara**—The epiphysis fuses in displaced position resulting in coxavara.
2. **AVN**—May develop due to forceful manipulation. Use of threaded pins in place of bulky nails reduces the incidence of AVN.
3. **Chondrolysis**—Develop following reduction. Joint space is reduced and hip becomes stiff. Postreduction rest reduces the incidence of Chondrolysis.
4. **OA**—Occurs if the slippage is not reduced. AVN predisposes to early secondary complication.

Perthes disease

Also known as coxa plana or osteochondritis of femoral capital epiphysis. It is a noninflammatory self-limiting condition that heals with flattening on weight bearing surface of femoral head.

During fourth month of the intrauterine life, the femoral head derives its blood supply from the nutrient artery, circumflex femoral artery and arteries accompanying ligamentum teres. The supply by the nutrient artery gradually declines and almost disappears by 7 years of age. Then the femoral head depends entirely upon the circumflex femoral artery. In case of joint effusion due to trauma, nonspecific synovitis or transient synovitis, increase in the intraarticular pressure compresses the circumflex femoral arteries compromising the circulation to femoral head and AVN [11].

Causes

The exact cause is not known. Male are more affected than female (4:1 ratio). Age of onset is about (2–12) years, mean age (4–8) years. In about 12% of cases, bilateral involvement is present. There is transient avascularity to the growing femoral head either due to thrombosis, synovitis, trauma resulting in AVN. It is followed by revascularization, reabsorption of the necrotic bone and lying down of the new bones. The disease process lasts for 2–4 years.

Pathogenesis

The disease process involves part or whole of the capital femoral epiphysis. The articular cartilage is normal. The early sign in X-ray shows increased density of femoral head due to disuse osteoporosis of the femoral head. There is gradual revascularization with lying down of new bone over dead trabeculae resulting in true increase in density. Microscopic examination reveals pronounced necrosis of the bone is grossly distorted. Bone marrow trabeculae and the bone fragments are soft in consistency. Later the X-ray shows area of increased density interspersed with area of radiolucent i.e., the bone appears to be fragmented. The radiolucent area represents dead bones and dense area represents lying down of new bones. The femoral head may be distorted, flattened, and extruded laterally. Gradually the femoral head regain its homogenous density over a period of 2–4 years. In the mean time, it may lose its density or sphericity. Ultimate shape of head is important as the prognosis and joint condition depends on it. If the head remain spherical even if its size is spherical the prognosis is good. Loss of spherical shape predisposes to early secondary OA.

The disease process is divided into **three stages**.

- **Stage 1**—Part or whole of the bony head of the femur is affected. It still looks normal on X-ray. There is synovitis and joint space may be increased
- **Stage 2**—The trabeculae on the dead bone may be fractured. Sometimes a subchondral fracture is seen on X-ray. Ingrowth of the new blood vessels and lying down on the new bones on the dead trabeculae occur. The metaphysis becomes hyperemic.
- **Stage 3**—With the lying down of new bones the dead bones are reabsorbed. Shape of the head depends on its management. Eventually normal density of the head is restored.

Clinical features

Insidious onset of pain, which is intermittent in nature. The child limps while walking and running. In the absence of symptoms and with minimal symptoms gross X-ray changes may be seen. The age of onset is 4–8 years. The condition is more common in boys than in girls with 4:1 ratio.

Wasting of the glutei may be present. In the early stage, the joint is irritable, so all the movement is reduced and painful. Overtime the joint irritability is reduced and almost all the movements return to normal except abduction-internal rotation.

Investigations

X-ray: Before the disease become apparent in X-ray, CT scan is diagnostic. Early stage there is apparent increase in density due to disuse osteoporosis of the neck and increased joint space.

Flattening, fragmentation, and lateral displacement of epiphysis with rarefaction and widening of metaphysis is seen in the later stage [12]. Depending on the involvement, the X-ray changes vary. Extent of involvement varies with the age of the child and stage of the disease. There are **four grades.**

- **Grade 1**—Anterior portion of head is involved. There is no collapse of the involved segment. No metaphyseal or epiphyseal plate involvement. Healing occurs without any significant effect.
- **Grade 2**—More is the involvement. Still enough part of the head remains viable to prevent collapse. Metaphyseal changes may be seen but no epiphyseal involvement.
- **Grade 3**—one-third of the femoral head is involved. Both metaphyseal and epiphyseal plate are involved, so prognosis is poor.
- **Grade 4**—The entire femoral capital epiphysis is involved. Both metaphysis and epiphysis plate and growth plate are involved. The head collapses and prognosis is poor.

Management

Management of Perthes disease depends on the severity of the disease. Grade 1 and 2 are kept under supervision. Early the limitation of the movement, poor is the prognosis. Therefore, maintenance or restoration of the full hip ROM is the aim of physiotherapy management.

During the irritable stage, bed rest with traction for about 3 weeks is given.

The ultimate aim of management is to maintain the sphericity of the head of the femur and to maintain or restore JROM.

Head of the femur must be contained well inside the acetabulum, so that the acetabulum will mold the head without distortion. The femoral head can be contained by abducting and internal rotating the hip. It can be achieved either by plaster cast (broom stick cast) or by splint [13]. To allow amputation with the hip joint contain hip abduction orthosis with trilateral socket is suitable.

The ischial seat present on the posterior wall of the line of socket. The ischial tuberosity (IT) rests on standing. The thigh remains in abduction with the foot off the ground resting on a splint. From the trilateral socket, another vertical bar with rocker bottom transmits the body weight from the IT to the ground.

If containment can't be achieved due to limitation of hip abduction range, give bed rest and traction; gradually abduct the limb to attain containment.

Surgically varus osteotomy of the femur or innominate osteotomy of the pelvis is followed by hip spica immobilization for 4—6 weeks.

Grade 1 needs no treatment. Ensure that the hip JROM is maintained. **Grade 2** should be kept under supervision and maintain full hip JROM. **Grade 3** under 7 years of age also kept under supervision, above 7 years of age requires containment. Earlier is the onset better is the prognosis as more growth potential is left for remodeling. **Grade 4** at all ages need containment.

Piriformis syndrome

The piriformis syndrome refers to pain associated with tightness or spasm of the piriformis muscle that puts pressure on the underlying sciatic nerve, causing radicular symptoms. The symptoms can be aggravated by stretching or contracting the piriformis, that is, by medially rotating the hip passively to stretch the muscle or by resisting lateral rotation, causing the piriformis to contract. The clinician uses these passive or resisted movements to elicit the patient's symptoms and to identify piriformis syndrome. Piriformis is a strong external rotator of the hip in extension and abductor of hip in flexion. They are small but very strong hip external rotator whereas there is no muscle around the hip whose primary action is internal rotation. Therefore, muscle imbalance develops between hip internal and external rotators. The hip tends to be externally rotated almost in all positions. The gluteus medius & minimus are capable of medial rotation of the hip, particularly when the hip is flexed. The gluteus maximus and piriformis also may contribute to medial rotation of the hip when the hip is flexed. Some of the hip adductors may generate small medial rotation moments, but their contributions are small and variable. Another muscle described as a medial rotator of the hip is the tensor fasciae latae. The medial hamstrings, the semimembranosus, and semitendinosus also exhibit small medial rotation moment arms with the hip in extension. These data reveal that the muscles that medially rotate the hip depend on hip position and are intimately related to the function of the knee. The most common functional use of active medial rotation of the hip occurs during the stance phase of gait when the pelvis rotates over the fixed femur and as the hip moves from the flexed to the extended position. During this period, the abductors contract to support the pelvis in the frontal plane, and the hamstrings are supporting the hip and knee in the sagittal plane. Their activity in medial rotation demonstrates an efficient use of muscles to perform simultaneous tasks.

Unlike the other actions of the hip, there are no muscles at the hip whose primary and consistent action is medial rotation of the hip.

Inactive gluteal muscles facilitate development of piriformis syndrome. In sitting positions, gluteal become inactive due to over active hip flexors as per the reciprocal innervations principle [14]. It leads to over activity of piriformis, which is synergist to gluteal. Since, most of the time, we adapt sitting posture, hypertrophy of the piriformis predisposes to piriformis syndrome.

Stiffness/hypomobility of SI joint, result in abnormal GAIT pattern and malfunction of the piriformis leading to P.S. In case of overpronated foot, piriformis overacts to prevent excessive medial rotation of the tibia predisposing to piriformis syndrome.

Protective spasm of the piriformis almost in all the cases of sciatica as sciatic nerve passes underneath the piriformis results in impaired circulation → ischemia and necrosis → necrosed muscle fiber are replaced by fibrous tissue, which contract over time giving rise to piriformis syndrome.

Clinical features—Complains of pain and tenderness on the buttock and sciatica like pain. Pain aggravates in standing and walking. The symptoms of P.S often become worse after prolonged walking or running/sitting. One may feel better on lying on back.

Hip internal rotation, adduction with hip flexed to about 60° range will be decreased. Piriformis tendon can be seen/palpated in side lying on contralateral side at the edge of the bed with affected hip flexed to 60°, adducted, knee flexed, and foot behind the opposite leg on the lateral aspect, proximal to greater trochanter.

Piriformis syndrome is diagnosed on clinical basis by ruling out other possible conditions of L-spine and SI joint.

Piriformis sign—In relaxed supine lying position, observe both the foot from foot end of the bed. The involved L/E is relatively externally rotated characterized by excessive out-toeing.

Fair test—Patient in side lying on the sound side at edge of bed with affected hip adducted in 60° of flexion and knee out of the bed in flexion and foot behind the opposite knee. Therapist stands on the front, fixes the pelvis by one hand, and abducts the thigh by other hand placed on the knee. Pain on lateral aspect of buttock indicates test is positive. In the same position, resisted abduction may reproduce postero-lateral buttock pain along with radiation on L/L. Neural mobility may be impaired.

Management—Stretching of piriformis—U/L hip adduction in 60° of flexion, either in supine or side lying position by fixing the pelvis. B/L stretching is more effective as the pelvis can be fixed securely. In prone lying, hip internal rotation with knee flexed to 90°. In supine lying B/L hip adduction with the thighs crossed.

- Strengthening of hip internal rotators'
- Postural correction
- Correction of pronated foot
- Modalities includes ultrasound—frequency 1 MHz continuous mode.
- DTFM in side-lying position by the bend elbow can also be given.

Technique—Prepare the patient with undressing the part in side lying position, identify the correct spot, to and fro movement across the whole width of the muscle with adequate sweep and adequate pressure is applied so as to reach at the piriformis muscle. Therapist's olecranon process and patient's skin move as one single unit at a rate of 2–3 cycles per second. At the beginning patient may feel mild to moderate tenderness, over time as the discomfort subsides, increase the pressure. Duration -10 to 15 min.

Caution—Increased tenderness, Poor nutritional status of the skin, long term high dose steroid.

Effects—Mobilization of the fiber from its fellow fibers, disperse the nociceptive substances from the local site, local hyperaemia, local anesthesia, mechanoceptor stimulation, etc.

MET-Lewit's (1985) postisometric relaxation [15] — The hypertonic muscle is taken, to a length just short of pain or to a point where the resistance to the movement is first noted. At the motion barrier, the point gently contracts the hypertonic muscles for about 5—10 s, while the effort is resisted by the therapist with equal and oppositely directed counterforce. One can inhale during the effort. The amount of muscle contraction is minimal, about 10%—20% of maximum voluntary contraction, so that, the maneuver is never allowed to develop into a context of strength between the therapist and patient. After the effort, the patient is asked to exhale and relax completely. Only when complete relaxation is achieved, the muscle is taken to a new barrier gently w/o any stretch; otherwise, activation of stretch reflex may be counterproductive. Starting from the new barrier, the procedure is repeated for two to three time. To facilitate the process, muscles contraction may be combined with inhalation and relaxation with exhalation.

The classic stretch for the piriformis muscle is hip flexion with adduction and medial rotation even though research shows that in hip flexion the piriformis is a medial rotator. Research suggests that sitting with the knees crossed combining hip flexion with adduction and lateral rotation applies a significant stretch to the piriformis.

One should avoid prolong sitting, keeping the wallet on the back pocket.

Peripheral nerve injury about hip

Sciatic nerve (L4 to S3) is most commonly affected around pelvis/upper femur due to posterior hip dislocation. It results in paralysis of hamstrings along with other muscles below knee can be affected. Muscle atrophy present. The person walks with high steppage gait and finds inability to stand on heel or toes. There is sensory alteration in entire foot except the instep and medial malleolus.

Sciatic nerve may also be injured around the hip joint due to compression by piriformis as seen in cases of piriformis syndrome. It is characterized by pain and weakness of hip abduction and lateral rotation, pain on passive medial rotation of extended hip (FREIBERG SIGN) [16], burning pain and hyperesthesia (sacral/gluteal region as well as in sciatic nerve distribution). Medial rotation with flexion accentuates the problem.

Superior gluteal nerve (L4-S1) may be compressed as it passes between the piriformis and inferior border of gluteus minimus. It also gets injured during hip surgery. It results in acute gluteal pain that increases with ambulation, weakness of hip abductors and tenderness present just lateral to greater sciatic notch.

Femoral nerve (L2-L4) may be compressed during child birth, anterior dislocation of femur, trauma during hernia surgery, stripping of varicose vein, hip surgery or fracture. It results in inability to flex the thigh on trunk, extend the knee, wasting of quadriceps, loss of sensation over medial aspect of distal thigh and medial aspect of leg and foot.

Obturator nerve (L2-L4) may be compressed as it leaves the pelvis and enter the leg in the obturator tunnel caused by pelvic or hip surgery, obstetric palsy during pregnancy, fracture, and tumors. It results in groin pain from symphysis pubis to medial aspect of knee, sensory deficit over middle medial part of thigh, hip adduction, flexion, lateral rotation also affected.

Meralgia paresthetica

Pain, paresthesias, and sensory loss over anterolateral aspect of thigh due to entrapment of lateral cutaneous nerve of the thigh (LCNT) is referred as meralgia paresthetica (MP). It is also known as Bernhardt-Roth syndrome [17]. The LCNT is branch of the lumbar plexus (L1−L3). It functions primarily as a sensory nerve. The LCNT then emerges at the lateral border of the psoas major, crosses the iliacus, to the anterior superior iliac spine. The nerve then passes under the inguinal ligament and over the sartorius muscle and enters the thigh as it divides into an anterior and posterior branch.

MP occurs when the lateral femoral cutaneous nerve—which supplies sensation to the surface of your outer thigh—becomes compressed, or pinched. The lateral femoral cutaneous nerve is purely a sensory nerve and doesn't affect your ability to use your leg muscles.

In most people, this nerve passes through the groin to the upper thigh without trouble. But in MP, the lateral femoral cutaneous nerve becomes trapped—often under the inguinal ligament, which runs along your groin from your abdomen to your upper thigh.

Grossman et al. classified MP as being idiopathic or iatrogenic with a subclassification of idiopathic as mechanical or metabolic [18].

Idiopathic: Mechanical factors can result in compression of the LCNT along its anatomical course. MP has been related to the following factors: obesity (BMI ≥30), pregnancy, tight garments such as jeans, corset, military armor and police uniforms, seat belts, direct trauma, muscle spasm, scoliosis, iliacus hematoma, and leg length changes. Metabolic factors reported include diabetes mellitus, alcoholism, and lead poisoning. Being overweight or pregnancy can increase the pressure on your lateral femoral cutaneous nerve, Nerve injury due to diabetes or seat belt injury after a motor vehicle accident, Repeated leg motions (long periods of biking, walking, squatting) also can lead to MP. Scar tissue near the inguinal ligament due to injury/surgery may cause MP.

Iatrogenic: MP has also been reported as a post-surgical complication after hip joint replacement through anterior approach and posterior lumbar spine surgery. When the patient is prone the anterior hip gets compressed from the surgical equipment utilized during surgery, which led to the onset of MP. MP has also been reported, to a lesser extent, as a post-surgical complication in iliac bone harvesting, open and laparoscopic appendectomy, cesarean with epidural analgesics, and obstetric and gynecological surgery.

People between the ages of 30 and 60 are at a higher risk.

Clinical features: Patients may complain of burning type of pain, numbness, muscle aches, coldness, in their lateral or anterolateral aspect of thigh. The symptoms may vary from mild pain without interfering the functions to severe that limits functions. Factors aggravating the symptoms are standing, walking, whereas sitting relieves the symptoms.

Pelvic compression test: The pelvic compression test was first described by Nouraei et al. in 2007 [19]. The patient is in side lying position on opposite side. Apply downward compression force to the pelvis and maintains pressure for 45 s. If the patient reports an alleviation of symptoms, the test is considered positive. A downward force to the innominate will relax the inguinal ligament and temporarily alleviate the patient's symptoms.

Neurodynamic testing: Butler's Neurodynamic test for adverse mechanical tension of the LCNT is performed in side lying position on opposite side with hip and knee bend. Therapist stands behind and stabilizes the pelvis by one hand, with the other hand bend the knee and adduct the thigh. The test is said to be positive if the original symptom is reproduced that aggravates with neck flexion and relieves with neck extension suggestive of adverse neural tension for LCNT.

Tinel's sign: Tap along the course of the LCNT on the anterior aspect of thigh, if the original symptom is reproduced the Tinel's sign is said to be positive.

Investigations: Neurophysiological studies such as somatosensory evoked potentials (81.3% sensitivity) and sensory nerve conduction (65.2% sensitivity), MRI are diagnostic of LCNT.

Physicians also choose to conduct a nerve block test (using 1% Lidocaine) at the site where the LCNT exits the pelvis at the inguinal ligament; approximate site of injection is 1 cm medial and inferior to the ASIS or at the point of maximum pain. The test is considered positive if the patient has immediate symptom relief that lasts 30–40 min after the injection.

Management

Avoid use of tight garment, belt, corset, etc. Wearing loose clothing, losing excess weight, avoiding compression activities are recommended.

Medical treatment for MP often includes the use of NSAIDS, Corticosteroid injections, Tricyclic antidepressants, Gabapentin, pulsed radiofrequency ablation using a high-frequency alternating current and LCNT nerve block using a combination of Lidocaine and corticosteroids.

Physical therapy include Active Release Techniques (ART), mobilization/manipulation for the pelvis, myofascial therapy for the rectus femoris and illiopsoas, transverse friction massage of the inguinal ligament, stretching exercises for the hip and pelvic musculature, and pelvic stabilization/abdominal core exercise. Low impact aerobics, brisk walking, swimming, cycling etc may be encouraged. Transcutaneous electrical nerve stimulation is effective in the treatment of painful peripheral neuropathy like MP. Neurostimulation techniques including transcranial magnetic stimulation and cortical electrical stimulation, spinal cord stimulation, and deep brain stimulation have also been found effective in the treatment of neuropathic pain as MP.

Surgical interventions: LCNT neurolysis and resection are optional interventions in cases where non-surgical management has failed.

Clinical reasoning

The clinical reasoning process acts as a filter whereby many possibilities are reduced to the most probable. Frequently, inexperienced clinicians use little information to reach a diagnosis. In contrast, the experienced clinician uses multiple impairment variables to establish clinical patterns which should correlate with the events leading up to the pain as well as the consequences of the pain. By reducing the variables into pattern recognition, the experienced clinician can use inductive and deductive reasoning to confirm their "working hypothesis." When the clinical features do not fit a known pattern, then deductive reasoning is used to examine the basics, correlate this with principles of patho-anatomy, biomechanics, and neurophysiology to form a management strategy for the new clinical pattern. Importantly, the subjective examination and disability measures should correlate with the physical examinations impairment measures, which in turn should be used to assess the outcomes of treatment. In this manner the efficacy, and hence validity and reliability of each and every technique can be assessed.

Clinical reasoning for posterior hip pain

The diagnosis and management of posterior hip pain have continued to evolve because of an increase in understanding of hip biomechanics and clinical anatomy and availability of treatment options. The hip has an intimate biomechanical relationship with the spine and lower limbs and an anatomic proximity with intrapelvic and extrapelvic structures.

Patients presenting with intra- or extraarticular posterior hip pain require an ordered history and physical examination with specific diagnostic tests to assess all structures comprising or around the hip. These structures may be categorized as osseous, capsule-labral, musculo-tendinous, or neurovascular, or as part of the kinematic chain.

The human body works as a unit, and any change in the normal range of motion of a joint could lead to compensatory changes both proximal and distal to that given joint. The complex biomechanics require a balanced interaction between anatomic structures, neuromuscular activity, and range of motion.

Posterior hip pain can occur from intraarticular or extraarticular sources or a combination of both sources. The history and physical examination, complemented by imaging studies and ancillary tests, including intraarticular injection, are critical in defining the origin of the patient's pain.

Precise diagnosis is key to directing both nonsurgical and surgical interventions for intra- and extraarticular hip pathologies. The main differential diagnoses are intraarticular hip pathologies such as posterior femoro-acetabular impingement (FAI), hip-spine syndrome, intrapelvic or extrapelvic sciatic entrapment, pudendal nerve entrapment, ischio-femoral impingement (IFI), hamstrings origin tendinopathy, and deep gluteal syndrome.

In addition to malfunction of anatomic structures, biomechanical alterations around the hip are also an important factor that causes pain. Interest in hip anatomy has led to the knowledge of subtle abnormalities in the orientation of the femoral neck or the lesser trochanter (LT) leading to extraarticular hip impingement, kinematic chain disturbances such as a load transfer due to hip extension block, and posterior hip pain.

A cadaver study performed by Kivlan et al. showed that the greater trochanter can impinge on the ischium during a combination of hip flexion, abduction, and external rotation [20]. This phenomenon has also been described as greater trochanteric pelvic impingement. Limitations in range of motion due to an impingement can lead to adaptations in lumbo-pelvic kinematics. A biomechanical study by Popovich et al. supported the clinical finding that pelvic inclination may play a role in increasing loads on the lumbar spine [21]. Another cadaver biomechanical study by Gómez-Hoyos J proved a notable relationship between simulated IFI and lumbar facet load changes during terminal hip extension compared with native hips [22]. Limited terminal hip extension due to simulated IFI significantly increases L3-4 and L4-5 lumbar facet joint load when compared with non-IFI native hips.

Hip problems such as flexor contracture, posterior acetabular overcoverage, and femoral retroversion can also limit terminal hip extension. Hip joint disorders that limit terminal hip extension may give rise to low back pain due to hyper-lordosis, narrowing of the foramina, and consequent lumbar nerve root compression, facet joint overload. Therefore, every hip examination should include a back examination and every back examination a hip examination.

Sciatic nerve kinematic adaptations and irritation can also occur as a result of dynamic narrowing of the ischial tunnel in posterior hip impingement. The sciatic nerve exits the pelvis through the sciatic notch and has notable mobility with hip movement. Coppieters et al. found that the sciatic nerve has 28 mm of excursion during hip flexion. However, this motion may be affected by piriformis penetration of the sciatic nerve occurring in 16.2% of the population as well as other etiologies, such as abnormal nerve anatomy.

As the hip moves into deep flexion, abduction, and external rotation, the sciatic nerve glides across the posterior border of the greater trochanter. This observation is key to understanding rehabilitation and maintenance of mobility in patients with sciatic nerve disorders.

In the full-flexed, abducted, and externally rotated state, the semimembranosus muscle origin and the posterior edge of the greater trochanter can come into contact. In addition, a spiraling phenomenon of the sciatic nerve has also been observed during flexion and abduction of the hip and may explain the relief of sciatic nerve strain. Chronic hamstring origin abnormalities have been described in patients with posterior hip impingement in approximately 50% of cases. However, other mechanisms should also be considered. Most hamstring injuries occur after indirect trauma resulting from overuse, excessive stretching, or forceful contraction leading to avulsion or muscle strains and tears. Patients with hamstring tears, regardless of the cause, can experience sciatic nerve irritation and symptoms in the lower buttock because of inflammation and the presence of scar tissue. This condition, known as hamstring syndrome, is an important differential diagnosis in patients with posterior hip pain.

In a cadaver study, Miller and Webb found that the sciatic nerve has an intimate relationship with the ischium and the hamstring origin [23]. The sciatic nerve was located at an average of 1.2 ± 0.2 cm from the most lateral aspect of the IT. Branches of the sciatic nerve can also be irritated, and aberrant branches can be identified. The branches to the long head of the biceps femoris and semitendinosus muscle emerge near the IT (6.9 and 7.1 cm, respectively).

Posterior hip pain originates mainly from extraarticular conditions causing a more global pain distribution and radiation. By contrast, disorders from inside the joint radiate to the anterior or medial thigh as the femoral or obturator nerves innervate most of the intraarticular hip.

A standardized clinical evaluation allows for the identification of intraarticular and extraarticular pathologies. In all cases of posterior hip pain, the first step must be to rule out spinal involvement based on patient history and physical examination and/or MRI, if necessary. The most efficient order of examination starts with standing tests, followed by seated, supine, lateral, and finally, prone tests. A complete physical examination is performed. The location of the reported pain is a valuable guide to assist in a correct diagnosis.

Palpation of the gluteal structures is fundamental for the diagnosis of posterior hip pain. Using the IT as a reference for palpation, the reproduction of pain can guide the probable source of symptoms. Pudendal nerve entrapment is considered with pain on palpation medial to the IT. Hamstring tendon pathologies are possible with palpation pain lateral or posterior to the IT. IFI is considered with palpation pain lateral to the IT; entrapment of the sciatic nerve at this location is termed hamstring syndrome. Deep gluteal syndrome is characterized by pain superolateral to IT at the sciatic notch. Pain around the ischium can be explained by a number of causes that increase or decrease pain, and the presence of radiated pain. Pudendal nerve pain is mainly located medial to the ischium and worsens with sitting (although is alleviated when sitting on a toilet or a donut pillow), decreases on standing, is absent on walking, but progressively worsens throughout the day.

Pudendal nerve entrapment can produce burning, tearing, stabbing lightning-like, electrical, sharp shooting, and/or foreign body sensations. Changes in skin sensation around the pudendal nerve area can also be present.

Hamstrings issues and IFI can often coexist. Patients presenting with chronic hamstring injury have subtle neural issues exacerbated by walking and sitting pain with active contractions.

IFI is associated with low back pain and long-stride walking pain. Pain lateral to the ischium during the toe-off/preswing phase of gait (i.e., hip in terminal extension) could be associated with IFI, in which the LT rubs the lateral border of the ischium or the semimembranosus tendon origin. In contrast, pain lateral to the ischium during heel strike when the hip is flexed and the hamstrings contracted could be associated with hamstring origin injuries.

Pain during both phases of gait could also be present as abnormalities of the hamstring origin have been found in 50% of the patients with IFI. Similar to IFI, the greater trochanter could be involved in posterior hip pain. An abnormal contact between the posterior aspect of the greater trochanter and the ischium can produce pain and sciatic nerve irritation during flexion-abduction-external rotation (i.e., greater trochanteric pelvic/sciatic nerve impingement). Patients with sciatic nerve entrapment often present with a traumatic mechanism of injury, inability to sit 30 min in a balanced position, and radiating pain down the ipsi-lateral leg. Patients may also present with other neurologic symptoms, such as abnormal reflexes or weakness.

Sacroiliac (SI) joint dysfunction, hamstring tears, and intraarticular hip pathology may mimic sciatic nerve entrapment by presenting symptoms such as aching, burning sensation, or cramping in the buttock or posterior thigh.

Sitting pain with balanced sitting avoidance is usually associated with sciatic nerve entrapment beneath the piriformis muscle.

Martin et al. proved that the combination of the seated piriformis stretch test with the piriformis active test has a sensitivity of 91% and a specificity of 80% for the endoscopic finding of sciatic nerve entrapment [24]. When both tests are negative, extrapelvic sciatic nerve entrapment at the piriformis muscle is unlikely.

A history of pain inferior and medial to the posterior superior iliac spine suggests SI joint disorders. This finding is even more helpful in the absence of lumbar pain. Only 4% of patients with SI joint pain mark any pain above L5 on self-reported pain drawings. Dreyfuss et al. established that SI joint tenderness has the highest sensitivity (89%). Although the specificity is low, this feature may serve as a reasonable screening test for SI joint problems, differentiated by palpation of the gluteus maximus origin tendinitis. The Patrick flexion, abduction, external rotation (FABER); axial and lateral compression; and Gaenslen tests help to determine extension and flexion SI strain, or pain. Pathologies that produce a loss of hip extension, such as IFI and shortened anterior hip capsule/quadriceps muscles, can cause SI joint pain.

Intrapelvic or extrapelvic structures could also produce pudendal nerve entrapment and/or sciatic nerve issues. A focused urologic and gynecologic history is obtained to detect any symptoms suggestive of intrapelvic entrapment, such as cyclic variations in pain (i.e., endometriosis, normal menstruation). Painful intercourse and bladder or bowel issues, such as incontinence, can also help identify intrapelvic disorders as the source of the pain.

Causes of intraarticular posterior hip pain have been described. Patients with posterior labral tears report a variety of mechanical symptoms, including clicking, locking, catching, or giving way, mainly during hip extension. Posterior labral cysts produced from labral tears can also irritate the sciatic nerve.

Long-stride walking test is intended to provoke impingement between the LT and ischium during extension of the hip. The test is positive if the posterior pain is reproducible and the patient grabs the affected hip lateral to the ischium (as shown in the picture) during extension, whereas pain is alleviated when walking with short strides or abducted hips.

Clinical reasoning for lateral hip pain

Primary area of pain is directly over right GT. This pain could extend approximately 75% of the distance down the lateral thigh to the knee, and sometimes in sitting with the knees crossed the pain would extend more posterior to the greater trochanter. Pain is aching in nature, although sometimes it feels hot, burning sensations. Tenderness over left GT, but it does not cause any functional problem. At night one finds difficulty, lying on either side. Lying supine is comfortable, but it is difficult to maintain it whole night. One often wakes up with pain. Pain fluctuates depending on the positions one adopts or activities he/she perform. Hip and thigh pain is aggravated by sitting particularly with the affected leg crossed, and also deep sitting as in squatting. Walking at a fast pace on uneven terrains and up hills, stairs and climbing ladders are also provocative of symptoms. It suggests the most likely pain source is to be gluteal tendinopathy, trochanteric bursitis or iliotibial band syndrome (ITB).

The key features that fit this pattern are pain and tenderness directly over the greater trochanter with pain aggravation on direct compression (lying on this side), passive compression associated with hip adduction, that is, side-lying with the affected side uppermost, sitting with right leg crossed and combinations of compressive and tensile load, that is, walking at fast pace or on uneven terrain; climbing stairs, hills and ladders. It is, however, common for patients with local soft tissue pathology at the greater trochanter to complain of pain that extends to the knee and radiates around the greater trochanter.

Following the subjective questioning, it is evident that the lumbar spine would also need to be assessed to rule out lumbar spine as the source of lateral thigh pain. Pain extending to the foot or the presence of pins and needles or numbness would raise suspicion of a spinal or neurogenic origin. The aching nature of pain is usually consistent with symptomatic gluteal tendinopathy. Hot and burning type of pain description often indicates a neurogenic origin.

A gradual worsening over time suggests that the load across the tendon may have been suboptimal, leading to a gradual decline in load tolerance. Walking hills is more challenging for the lateral stability mechanism of the hip and pelvis. One lives in a hilly area, and all of his/her walking involved this higher-level challenge for which gluteal tendons are evidently no longer optimally adapted. In response to the first signs of load failure, one does not reduce the load and continue to walk through the pain and with purposefully long strides, which may amplify the loads across the lateral hip during stance phase.

Standing posture with anteriorly translated pelvis relative to the ankles and shoulders, resulting in a relatively extended hip position with the center of mass of the trunk falling posterior to the hip joint increases load at the anterior hip, and one appeared to respond to that load by increasing the activity of his/her tensor fascia lata (TFL) muscles. The patient is asked what standing postures he/she tends to adopt while at work or at social functions because the posture a patient displays when under examination by a health professional may not be truly indicative of the patient's habitual standing posture, particularly during prolonged standing. One spends a considerable amount of time on his/her feet at work. Natural resting posture often involves 'hanging on one hip in adduction.

During the loading phase on the affected side in which the pelvis drops rapidly into a mild lateral tilt, followed by reproduction of lateral hip pain during the late stance phase. Inadequate pelvic control in the coronal plane was also demonstrated in other single leg loading tasks such as single leg stance and single leg squat where the pelvis laterally translated and tilted, resulting in excessive hip adduction. These tasks were assessed with the nonweight-bearing foot lifted off the ground behind, allowing only 10−20° of hip flexion on this side. It has been recommended that the nonweight-bearing hip should not be flexed more than 30° during assessment of these tasks [25] because the hip flexors on that side could be used to elevate the pelvis when maintained in higher ranges of hip flexion, and as a result, inadequate hip abductor function may be masked [25].

Trunk position should also monitor because lateral trunk flexion or shift brings the center of mass over the supporting foot, reducing the requirement for hip abductor activity, once again masking and compensating for hip abductor muscle dysfunction.

Gentle manual guidance into a more neutral posture immediately results in relaxation of the muscle tension suggests firstly that this tension was due to "active muscle holding" rather than passive soft tissue tightness and, secondly, that postural correction may be a beneficial strategy for reducing anterior hip loading and tension within the anterior aspect of the ITB. Tensioning of the ITB, whether passive due to joint positioning, active due to recruitment of inserting or adjacent musculature, or both, may increase compressive loads on the soft tissues at the greater trochanter and, if excessive, may influence tissue health and load tolerance.

Hanging on one hip in adduction is a common postural habit, and certainly everyone who stands in this manner does not develop symptomatic gluteal tendinopathy. Considered alone, this would not be considered diagnostic. However, in a clinical scenario, this postural habit is consistent with a pattern of abductor weakness or dysfunction that is typical of those with symptomatic gluteal tendinopathy.

More formal testing of hip abductor muscle function was performed through assessment of active lag of abduction and abductor strength. In their role as superficial abductors, TFL and upper gluteus maximus exert their effect via the ITB. They will be mechanically disadvantaged as the hip moves into inner range abduction and the ITB becomes relatively slack. The deeper abductors (gluteus medius and minimus) that exert their effect directly via the greater trochanter will then be primarily important for achieving movement through this inner range. Subsequently, loss of ability to move actively into inner-range abduction is likely to reflect deficiencies in these 'trochanteric abductors. Although active range may be limited by passive joint or soft tissue restriction, the lag measurement reflects the ability of the abductors to move the hip through its available passive range. One's active lag of abduction was over 20° on both sides but was slightly greater on the right, reflecting poor function of the trochanteric abductors on both sides. Normative data are not available in the literature; however, clinically those with normal function can usually lift the hip into an abduction range that is within 5—10° of their passive range. Deficits in hip abductor muscle strength in those with symptomatic gluteal tendinopathy have been demonstrated when compared with both the asymptomatic or less symptomatic hip and a pain-free control population [26]. One's abductor weakness and pain reproduction during strength testing was consistent with a diagnosis of gluteal tendinopathy and provided a treatment direction for the rehabilitation process.

Differential diagnosis: The main conditions to consider with such a presentation are gluteal tendinopathy, hip joint pathology and referred lumbar pain.

Lumbar spine examination: All active lumbar movements are full range and pain-free. No tenderness was elicited on lumbar spine palpation, with only mild hypomobility of the thoracolumbar region detected. Neurodynamic examination—straight leg raise is negative and of normal range.

Hip examination: Hip range of motion is normal and equal on both the sides. Both the quadrant (or scour) test and flexion adduction internal rotation (FADDIR) impingement test are negative. Other physical tests are selected for testing the hypothesis of painful gluteal tendinopathy, including sustained single leg stance; flexion, abduction, external rotation (FABER); flexion, adduction, external rotation—passive and resisted internal rotation (FADER); and hip adduction (passive and with resisted isometric abduction).

In reasoning a differential diagnosis, let's first consider referred lumbar spine pain: One described the hip pain as emanating from the region of the greater trochanter, rather than typical radicular pain, which would tend to emanate from the spine, extend across the buttock and then down the lateral thigh. The fact that there is no symptom past the knee and no pins and needles or numbness also reduced the likelihood of a primary lumbar issue. A burning feeling down the lateral aspect of thigh could suggest a neurogenic origin. All active lumbar movements are full and pain-free, straight leg raise is negative and of normal range and there is no tenderness on lumbar palpation, only some mild hypomobility of the thoracolumbar region. Based on these findings, the lumbar spine is considered an unlikely source of the lateral hip and thigh pain.

Second, hip joint pathology should be considered: Although lateral hip and thigh pain is commonly described by those with hip OA [27] localized pain over the greater trochanter is rarely the only or primary complaint in most clinical scenarios. Groin and posterior buttock pain are the most common types of pain associated with hip OA [28], or the patient may describe a pain which travels between the anterior and posterior hip, indicating this by grasping the hand around the lateral hip above the greater trochanter and below the ilium—referred to as the "C sign" [29]. Hip OA is also associated with loss of range of motion, particularly end-range flexion and internal rotation.

Acetabular labral tears may also produce hip pain in the absence of OA. The most common area of pain distribution is the anterior groin region, often extending down the anterior thigh to the knee [30]. Some patients with labral tears may experience buttock pain, and just over half complain of lateral hip pain [30]. An important clinical distinction here is that the lateral pain is not generally located over the greater trochanter but rather in the anterolateral hip region between the greater trochanter and the anterior superior iliac spine. Those with labral pathology may describe pain of an aching nature; however, many patients will also experience intermittent, sharp pain in the groin or anterolateral hip, most frequently with weight-bearing pivoting [31]. Mechanical descriptions such as catching, snapping, or locking are also common [31].

Physical tests, such as the quadrant or scour test and FADDIR, or impingement tests (flexion 90° + internal rotation) are very sensitive to the presence of intraarticular hip pathologies but have poor specificity [32]. Although the lack of specificity of such tests provides low confidence in determining the precise structural source of the pain when the test is positive, sensitive tests such as these are useful for ruling out a symptomatic pathology when the result is negative.

On physical examination, hip range of motion is normal and equal between sides, and scour and impingement tests are negative. These findings indicate that an intra-articular hip pain source is an unlikely contributor to the current pain state.

Lateral hip pain is reported to be most common in women aged over 40 years [33,34]. Pain and tenderness over the greater trochanter are considered hallmark signs of local soft tissue pathology [35]. The literature describes pain that is provoked particularly by side-lying, but also standing on one leg, walking up hills or stairs and moving to standing after prolonged sitting [36].

Traditionally referred to as trochanteric bursitis, it is now well established that gluteus medius and/or minimus tendinopathy is the most common pathology associated with lateral hip pain. However, there is often a coexistence of tendon and bursal changes, and even thickening of the ITB [37–40].

Physical tests do not accurately differentiate between these various pathologies but can be helpful in differentiating local soft tissue pathology from a more distant source, such as the spine or hip joint. Tenderness over the greater trochanter has been shown to be the most accurate test for predicting gluteal tendon changes on magnetic resonance imaging (MRI; highest proportion of true results, either positive or negative), with the lowest negative likelihood ratio, indicating that if palpation is negative on clinical testing, the result significantly increases the likelihood that the MRI will be negative too. However, the specificity of palpation findings is low, and the positive likelihood ratio is less useful, meaning that although the test is useful for ruling out tendinopathy when the trochanter is nontender, the trochanter may be tender in the absence of tendinopathy [41].

Palpation should then be used in combination with other tests that possess more useful positive likelihood ratios and positive predictive values. Physical tests, such as sustained single leg stance, FABER, FADER, and hip adduction (passive and with resisted isometric abduction), can be used to increase the likelihood of a diagnosis of gluteal tendinopathy when positive, particularly the tests that include an active muscle contraction (single leg stance; FADER with resisted isometric internal rotation; adduction with resisted isometric abduction) [41,42].

It is important to note, however, that many people without lateral hip pain have changes in their trochanteric tendons and bursae evident on MRI [38,41].

It is therefore important that radiological signs alone are not used for determining a pain source at the lateral hip. For a clinical diagnosis of symptomatic local soft tissue pathology at the lateral hip, the patient must be tender on palpation over the greater trochanter and be positive on at least one of the physical tests described. A positive test is defined as one that reproduces the patient's pain in the region of the greater trochanter.

Clinical reasoning for anterior hip pain

Anterior hip pain can result from upper lumbar spine, hip joint, iliopsoas tendinosis, iliopectineal bursitis, etc.

The hip joint is derived from L2 to S1 segments. Clinically, pain from hip joint pathology often experienced over L3 segment. Typically, patient with hip joint disease complains of pain midinguinal region that spreads over the front of thigh and knee and often confused as knee disorder. In case of hip joint pathology joint range of motion is limited in capsular pattern, that is, hip extension, internal rotation, abduction are limited and flexion limited to a lesser extent than extension. Pain and spasm over the referred pain zone, that is, quadriceps may limit knee flexion.

Iliopectineal bursa overlies the anterior aspect of the hip joint underneath the iliopsoas muscle. This bursa often communicates with the hip joint through the space between pubofemoral and iliofemoral ligaments. Hip joint effusion transmits into the bursa and results in anterior hip pain. Anterior hip pain due to hip arthritis, the hip joint range of motion is limited in capsular pattern. Iliopectineal bursitis, resisted hip flexion reproduces the original pain.

Pain radiating from the upper lumbar spine from which the lumbal plexus is derived in reproduced with lumbar spine movements and joint play. Pressure over the upper lumbar spine i.e., central PA, unilateral PA, transverse may reproduce the original symptoms and femoral nerve tension test may be positive. In prone position, bending the knee hurts the patient is suggestive of quadriceps shortening or positive femoral nerve tension test. Apply muscle energy technique (MET) to quadriceps by giving resisted isometric contraction at the end range. If MET, relaxes the muscle and improves the range, it is quadriceps tightness and the symptom aggravates in case of femoral nerve tension. Pain over the SI joint at end range of knee flexion is suggestive of SIJ dysfunction.

Femoral anteversion leads to increased ROM of internal rotation with a concomitant loss of external rotation which in turn affects pelvic rotation during activities such as ambulation. Increased adductor muscle tone results in anterior translation of the hip and anterior rotation of the ilium (hemi-pelvis) which results in counternutation, and "unlocking" of the SIJ. Torsion of the sacrum to the opposite side can place torsional load on the intervertebral disc between the fifth lumbar vertebrae and the sacrum.Cam and Pincer Lesions can occur in association with labral lesions [43]. A CAM lesion is the formation of extra bone on the head of the femur, whereas Pincer lesion is the formation of extra bone on the acetabular rim that overhangs the head & neck of femur. This extra bone that forms since birth may result in impingement with hip joint movement referred as FAI due to repetitive activity involving recurrent movement of the legs beyond the normal range of motion may cause hip impingement, which has been observed in certain athletes like football, baseball, soccer, tennis, hockey, lacrosse players, dancers, and golfers, etc. A bump forms on the edge of the femoral head that grinds the cartilage inside the acetabulum. The labrum can be crushed under the prominent rim of the acetabulum. In cases of Pincer impingement leading to labral tears. The evidence from the literature suggests that cam deformities develop in adolescents that are involved in sports that are subject to high rotational forces across the hip such as football and soccer. Cam deformities can lead to an increased risk of OA in later life. One complains of pain in the hip, groin and/or buttock. There is restriction of hip flexion beyond 90°. Pain aggravates with squatting, sitting in low chair, twisting activities such as cutting, pivoting, etc. Excessive tension in the external hip rotators can cause anterior acetabular impingement. Iliopsoas tendinosis may be associated with anterior labral lesions. Excessive anterior rotation of the innominate can cause anterior hip impingement.

X-rays and CT scan show bony abnormality of the femoral head, acetabular rim. MRI detects articular cartilage, labral damage. Pfirrmann et al. used MRI measurements of alpha angles and the depth of the acetabulum to determine the risk and incidence of CAM and Pincer lesions in the hip [44]. They concluded that a deep acetabulum and posteroinferior acetabular cartilage lesions were a characteristic finding of pincer impingement.

References

[1] Forst J, Forst C, Forst R, Heller KD. Pathogenetic relevance of the pregnancy hormone relaxin to inborn hip instability. Arch Orthop Trauma Surg 1997;116(4):209−12.

[2] Mirdad T. Incidence and pattern of congenital dislocation of the hip in Aseer region of Saudi Arabia. W Afr J Med 2002;21(3):218−22.

[3] Landa J, Benke M, Feldman DS. The limbus and the neolimbus in developmental dysplasia of the hip. Clin Orthop Relat Res 2008;466(4):776−81.

[4] Visser JD. Functional treatment of congenital dislocation of the hip. Acta Orthop Scand 1984;55(Suppl. 206):1−109.

[5] Gaillard F. Shenton line. Case study. Radiopaedia.org; 2008. https://doi.org/10.53347/rID-2711.

[6] Noordin S, Umer M, Hafeez K, Nawaz H. Developmental dysplasia of the hip. Orthop Rev 2010;2(2):e19.

[7] Sherk HH, Pasquariello Jr PS, Watters WC. Congenital dislocation of the hip. A review. Clin Pediatr 1981;20(8):513−20.

[8] Alkilaby AE, Alwash MJ. Preliminary over-head traction followed by closed reduction versus closed reduction without preliminary over-head traction; A comparative study discussing the treatment of developmental dysplasia of the hip (DDH) from the age of 6 to 24 months. Med J Babylon 2016;13(3):691−700.

[9] Rozkydal Z, Kovanda M. Chiari pelvic osteotomy in the management of developmental hip dysplasia: a long term follow-up. Bratisl Lek Listy 2003;104(1):7−13.

[10] Ucpunar H, Camurcu IY, Duman S, Ucpunar E, Sofu H, Bayhan AI. Obesity-related metabolic and endocrine disorders diagnosed during postoperative follow-up of slipped capital femoral epiphysis. Acta Orthop 2018;89(3):314−9.

[11] Liu B, Yi H, Zhang Z, Li Z, Yue D, Sun W. Association of hip joint effusion volume with early osteonecrosis of the femoral head. Hip Int 2012;22(2):179−83.

[12] Kruczynski J. Avascular necrosis of the proximal femur in developmental dislocation of the hip: incidence, risk factors, sequelae and MR imaging for diagnosis and prognosis. Acta Orthop Scand 1996;67(Suppl. 268):3−48.

[13] Kiepurska A. Late results of treatment in Perthes' disease by a functional method. Clin Orthop Relat Res 1991;272:76−81.

[14] Sherrington CS. On reciprocal innervation of antagonistic muscles − Tenth note. Proc Roy Soc Lond B 1907;79:337−49.

[15] Lewit K, Simons DG. Myofascial pain: relief by post-isometric relaxation. Arch Phys Med Rehabil 1984;65(8):452−6.

[16] Beatty RA. The piriformis muscle syndrome: a simple diagnostic maneuver. Neurosurgery 1994;34(3):512−4.

[17] Pearce JM. Meralgia paraesthetica (Bernhardt-Roth syndrome). J Neurol Neurosurg Psychiatry 2006;77(1):84.

[18] Cheatham SW, Kolber MJ, Salamh PA. Meralgia paresthetica: a review of the literature. Int J Sports Phys Ther 2013;8(6):883−93.

[19] Nouraei SA, Anand B, Spink G, O'Neill KS. A novel approach to the diagnosis and management of meralgia paresthetica. Neurosurgery 2007;60(4):696−700.

[20] Kivlan BR, Martin RL, Martin HD. Defining the greater trochanter-ischial space: a potential source of extra-articular impingement in the posterior hip region. J Hip Preserv Surg 2016;3(4):352−7.

[21] Popovich Jr JM, Welcher JB, Hedman TP, Tawackoli W, Anand N, Chen TC, Kulig K. Lumbar facet joint and intervertebral disc loading during simulated pelvic obliquity. Spine J 2013;13(11):1581—9.

[22] Gómez-Hoyos J, Schröder R, Reddy M, Palmer IJ, Martin HD. Femoral neck anteversion and lesser trochanteric retroversion in patients with ischiofemoral impingement: a case-control magnetic resonance imaging study. Arthroscopy 2016;32(1):13—8.

[23] Miller SL, Gill J, Webb GR. The proximal origin of the hamstrings and surrounding anatomy encountered during repair. A cadaveric study. J Bone Joint Surg Am 2007; 89(1):44—8.

[24] Martin HD, Reddy M, Gómez-Hoyos J. Deep gluteal syndrome. J Hip Preserv Surg 2015;2(2):99—107.

[25] Hardcastle P, Nade S. The significance of the Trendelenburg test. J Bone Joint Surg Br 1985;67(5):741—6.

[26] Allison K, Vicenzino B, Wrigley TV, Grimaldi A, Hodges PW, Bennell KL. Hip abductor muscle weakness in individuals with gluteal tendinopathy. Med Sci Sports Exerc 2016;48(3):346—52.

[27] Altman R, Alarcón G, Appelrouth D, Bloch D, Borenstein D, Brandt K, Brown C, Cooke TD, Daniel W, Feldman D, et al. The American cllege of rheumatology criteria for the classification and reporting of osteoarthritis of the hip. Arthritis Rheum 1991; 34(5):505—14.

[28] Lesher JM, Dreyfuss P, Hager N, Kaplan M, Furman M. Hip joint pain referral patterns: a descriptive study. Pain Med 2008;9(1):22—5.

[29] Byrd JW. Evaluation of the hip: history and physical examination. N Am J Sports Phys Ther 2007;2(4):231—40.

[30] Burnett RS, Della Rocca GJ, Prather H, Curry M, Maloney WJ, Clohisy JC. Clinical presentation of patients with tears of the acetabular labrum. J Bone Joint Surg Am 2006;88(7):1448—57.

[31] Tibor LM, Sekiya JK. Differential diagnosis of pain around the hip joint. Arthroscopy 2008;24(12):1407—21.

[32] Reiman MP, Thorborg K. Clinical examination and physical assessment of hip joint-related pain in athletes. Int J Sports Phys Ther 2014;9(6):737—55.

[33] Alvarez-Nemegyei J, Canoso JJ. Evidence-based soft tissue rheumatology: III: trochanteric bursitis. J Clin Rheumatol 2004;10(3):123—4.

[34] Segal NA, Felson DT, Torner JC, Zhu Y, Curtis JR, Niu J, Nevitt MC. Greater trochanteric pain syndrome: epidemiology and associated factors. Arch Phys Med Rehabil 2007;88(8):988—92.

[35] Hoffmann A, Pfirrmann CW. The hip abductors at MR imaging. Eur J Radiol 2012; 81(12):3755—62.

[36] Fearon AM, Scarvell JM, Neeman T, Cook JL, Cormick W, Smith PN. Greater trochanteric pain syndrome: defining the clinical syndrome. Br J Sports Med 2013;47(10): 649—53.

[37] Bird PA, Oakley SP, Shnier R, Kirkham BW. Prospective evaluation of magnetic resonance imaging and physical examination findings in patients with greater trochanteric pain syndrome. Arthritis Rheum 2001;44(9):2138—45.

[38] Blankenbaker DG, Ullrick SR, Davis KW, De Smet AA, Haaland B, Fine JP. Correlation of MRI findings with clinical findings of trochanteric pain syndrome. Skeletal Radiol 2008;37(10):903—9.

[39] Long SS, Surrey DE, Nazarian LN. Sonography of greater trochanteric pain syndrome and the rarity of primary bursitis. AJR Am J Roentgenol 2013;201(5):1083—6.

[40] Cowan RM, Ganderton CL, Cook J, Semciw AI, Long DM, Pizzari T. Does menopausal hormone therapy, exercise, or both improve pain and function in postmenopausal women with greater trochanteric pain syndrome? A 2 × 2 factorial randomized clinical trial. Am J Sports Med 2022;50(2):515—25.

[41] Grimaldi A, Mellor R, Nicolson P, Hodges PW, Bennell K, Vicenzino B. Utility of clinical tests to diagnose MRI-confirmed gluteal tendinopathy in patients presenting with lateral hip pain. Br J Sports Med 2016;51(6).

[42] Lequesne M, Mathieu P, Vuillemin-Bodaghi V, Bard H, Djian P. Gluteal tendinopathy in refractory greater trochanter pain syndrome: diagnostic value of two clinical tests. Arthritis Rheum 2008;59(2):241—6.

[43] Pun S, Kumar D, Lane NE. Femoroacetabular impingement. Arthritis Rheumatol 2015; 67(1):17—27.

[44] Pfirrmann CW, Duc SR, Zanetti M, Dora C, Hodler J. MR arthrography of acetabular cartilage delamination in femoroacetabular cam impingement. Radiology 2008; 249(1):236—41.

Index

Printed and bound by CPI Group (UK) Ltd, Croydon, CR0 4YY

08/05/2025

01864765-0002